CONTROL HIGH BLOOD PRESSURE
With and Without Medicine

Dr. Shahriar Mostafa
MBBS, MPH

ALL RIGHTS RESERVED

DEDICATION

I like dedicate this book to You, my reader

Thank you for taking an interest in this book. It's only for You, I get the inspiration to write another. You are giving me the opportunity to work on prevention of serious health conditions. Thank you for referring others to read this book. Thank you for overlooking my mistakes and giving your valuable time writing a review.

You are the cause of my improvement as a writer.

Contents

Introduction 9

Notes...11

PART ONE..12

What is Hypertension 13

Worldwide condition of Hypertension 15

Problems with uncontrolled hypertension 16

Cause of High Blood Pressure 17

Types of Hypertension 17

Symptoms of Hypertension 21

Risk factors for developing high blood pressure..........22

Diagnosis of Hypertension 26

Steps for Blood Pressure Measurement 26

Incorrect blood pressure measurement 29

24 hours Ambulatory blood pressure measurement (ABPM)......30

Choosing a device to measure Hypertension at home 32

How often should you visit your doctor?....................34

PART TWO..36

General Treatment Guideline for High Blood Pressure 37

Prehypertension 37

Stage 1 Hypertension...39

Stage 2 Hypertension...40

Stage 3 Hypertension...41

Lifestyle Modification to control hypertension 42

Modify your Diet 42

DASH Diet...43

Pritikin Diet 47

Exercise 50

Manage your weight...55

Medicines used in Hypertension..................................57

Diuretics 59

Beta-Blockers 62

Alpha-blockers for Hypertension 63

ACE inhibitors..65

Calcium Channel Blockers 67

Angiotensin II Receptor Blockers (ARB) 68

Direct Vasodilators..69

Central Agonists 70

Direct Renin Inhibitors 71

Peripheral-Acting Adrenergic Blockers 71

Medicine for Specific Conditions 72

Combination of medicine...73

Acupuncture for Hypertension 74

Natural or Herbal remedies for Hypertension 76

Hibiscus Tea for High Blood Pressure 77

Apple cider Vinegar for Hypertension.......................78

Garlic for Hypertension...79

Food supplements for hypertension.............................82

Coenzyme Q10 (CoQ10)...82

Omega-3 fatty acids 82

Amino Acids for Hypertension 83

Homeopathy for Hypertension 84

Meditation for Hypertension 85

PART THREE 87

What is hypertension...88

Which blood pressure Is more dangerous: systolic or diastolic? .88

Is isolated systolic pressure dangerous?....................88

Is hypertension inevitable?......................................89

Is Hypertension natural result of aging? 89

How to read blood pressure measurement? 90

Importance of monitoring blood pressure?................90

When should I start monitoring blood pressure? 91

What happens during 24-hour blood pressure monitoring? 91

Normal ambulatory blood pressure monitoring values? 92

Downside of ambulatory blood pressure monitoring................92

What is white coat Hypertension 93

What causes the white coat effect? 93

How will I know I have white coat hypertension? 94

What can I do about white coat hypertension?...........94

I have been diagnosed with high blood pressure, but could it be white coat hypertension? 94

Is white coat hypertension dangerous?.....................95

What is home blood pressure monitoring? 95

What Are the Complications Associated with Essential Hypertension?..96

What Is the Long-Term Outlook of hypertension? 97

Is hypertension a Result of Aging?..97

Is There Treatment for Prehypertension? 98

How excess salt may cause hypertension? 99

Are there any medicines that cause high blood pressure?..........99

How serious a risk is smoking for Hypertension? 100

How hypertension affects our brain? 100

What are the signs of Stroke?..101

Effect of hypertension on blood vessels? 102

Effect of hypertension on heart?...102

Is it right to use antihypertensive drugs every other day or 2 - 3 times per week?...103

When blood pressure Is high should I take an extra antihypertensive pill?...103

What must be done when blood pressure is too low? 104

Are sedatives tranquilizers effective in lowering blood pressure? 104

Oranges, coffee: do they really affect blood pressure levels?...105

Is there any cure for Hypertension? 105

In what level, should blood pressure be lowered with treatment? 105

When do, Hypertension need treatment...................................106

When should I call my doctor? 106

Job with Hypertension 107

How often should a hypertensive person visit the doctor?.......108

If hypertension runs in your family, would you get it too?........108

Does kosher or sea salt has an effect on hypertension? 109

Can you discontinue treatment if there are no symptoms?......109

Does wine have a positive effect on hypertension? 109

Is heart rate and blood pressure related? 110

Is Anxiety and Hypertension related?.....................................110

Are Recreational drugs with Hypertension dangerous? 111

What is the effect of Vape on hypertension? 111

How much Alcohol is safe with Hypertension?.........................111

What is the effect of hypertension on sex? 112

Can Erectile Dysfunction occur with Hypertension?.................113

Can Viagra be used with Hypertension? 114

Conclusion...116

Other Books by Dr. Shahriar Mostafa 117

Introduction

The one disease that will affect most of us is Hypertension. Hypertension is the medical name for High Blood Pressure (HBP). It is a disease of pandemic proportion effecting more and more people worldwide. HBP is the number 1 cause of heart attack and stroke, and it's poorly controlled worldwide. Recent World Health Report by World Health Organization (WHO) gives us an alarming information, it says "Overall, approximately 20% of the world's adults are estimated to have hypertension. The prevalence dramatically increases in patients older than 60 years: In many countries, 50% of individuals in this age group (60+) have hypertension. Worldwide, approximately 1 billion people have hypertension, contributing to more than 7.1 million deaths per year".

Hypertension is a disease of urbanization, it's a disease of lifestyle choice we make throughout our lives. So, we can change and modify our lifestyle to heal and prevent hypertension.

After we are diagnosed with hypertension, we face a common confusion. Our major concern becomes

- Should we use medicine to control Hypertension or control it only with lifestyle modification.
- What are the alternative treatments available and do they work.
- How good are the alternative treatments for hypertension without medicine.

We want to know

- Is there any preventable medicine for hypertension.
- Can we prevent it with diet and lifestyle modification.
- Are the medicines used to control hypertension safe in long term use.

In this book, I have tried to give all these answers. I have given pro and cons of drug and non-drug treatments used in hypertension. With information, I hope you can make an informed decision on your treatment plan. And you can also work on prevention of high blood pressure.

Before we begin a few words about me. By profession I am a doctor, completed my medical school 8 years back. Then I did a master's degree in public health (MPH). I have been working in a medical college hospital, treating patients and working on disease prevention for last 7 years. I write patient education books on diseases more than a year now, thanks to you I have two amazon bestselling books. Writing on diseases gives me the opportunity to reach a broad audience, it gives me opportunity to work on disease prevention on a larger scale.

Now about this book, there are lots of books on hypertension or High Blood pressure(HBP). The major difference of this book is, it is a small book. Our life has become busier than ever. With so much to see, learn and share we are always in short of time. It is difficult, sometimes unnecessary and time consuming to read a big book for information on blood pressure. This small book is packed with information that you will need. It is designed to save you a lot of time searching internet for information on hypertension. I have tried to keep the book as simple as possible and fun to read. You don't have to read it cover to cover, you can start anywhere using table of contents and finish it slowly.

Last part of this book includes answers some questions usually we want to ask about HBP but don't ask thinking it's silly or embarrassing.

Now let's see what is hypertension and how we can keep it controlled.

Happy reading.

Notes

Please remember, this book is not a prescription from a doctor. Do not change, increase, start or skip any ongoing treatment without consulting your doctor.

Every effort has been made to make this book as complete and as accurate as possible. However, there may be mistakes both typographical and in content. The opinion expressed in this book is personal opinion, diagnosis or treatment. You may disagree with the content. The statistical data presented in the book may be changed due to time or newer studies.

Therefore, this text should be used only as a general guide and not as the ultimate source of information.

The information provided here is medical information, learned from medical textbooks and journals and websites. As this is information on a specific disease you may already know some of them, but reading them once again will help you refresh what you know. And it will update your knowledge on high blood pressure with the latest data. All this information is also available on Internet. The book is designed to save time searching information.

Healthcare is ever changing, new data is added every year, new treatment emerges. This book will be updated every year. As you have purchased this book, I like to thank you and send you updates future editions free.

Please send me an email to dr.shahriar@doctor.com with "Hypertension " in subject line, so I can send you future editions of this ebook completely free.

PART ONE

HYPERTENSION OR HIGH BLOOD PRESSURE.

What is Hypertension

If you are a diagnosed patient of hypertension, then you already know what hypertension is. For those of us who still live life without high blood pressure, Hypertension is the medical term used for high blood pressure. We have a misconception that hypertension may be an indication of anxiety, tension, or hyperactive personality, but it does not indicate that.

Our body is an amazing piece of work. It's made up of trillions of cells. All these cells need food and oxygen to function. To provide food and oxygen to every cell we have a very efficient system. It is called the cardiovascular system. Cardiovascular system consists of heart, blood vessels and blood. Blood through veins and arteries carry and supply all the trillions of cells food and oxygen.

To move the blood inside our body we need a pump. Our heart is an efficient pump that pumps blood nonstop, from 3rd week after conception to all our life. Amazingly this small organ we call heart (average 11 ounces), pumps 2,000 gallons of blood through 60,000 miles of blood vessels nonstop every day.

This pumping action of the heart creates pressure. So, Blood Pressure (BP) is the force of the blood pushing against the inner walls of our blood vessels called arteries as it circulates throughout the body. For many reasons this pressure may increase from normal levels. When there is persistent Increased pressure, we call the condition Hypertension or High Blood Pressure.

The blood pressure reading is measured in millimeters of mercury (mmHg) There are two components of blood pressure reading:

- When the heart is constricting, or beating the pressure is highest. It is called SYSTOLIC pressure.
- And when the heart is relaxing between heartbeats the pressure is at its lowest point called DIASTOLIC pressure.

For example, a blood pressure reading is usually written or mentioned as 120/80 mmHg, or "120 over 80". Here SYSTOLIC pressure is 120 and the DIASTOLIC pressure is 80.

The problem with normal blood pressure is it depends on age and other factors. There is no absolute value that we can call normal. Usually the normal blood pressure for an adult age 20 or over is less than 120 systolic and less than 80 diastolic. Keep in mind Blood pressure rises with each heartbeat and falls when our heart relaxes between beats. It changes but in small level from minute to minute with changes in position, movement, exercise, stress or during sleep.

"The Joint National Committee on Prevention, Detection, Evaluation, and Treatment of High Blood Pressure has classified blood pressure measurements into several categories. According to this guideline;

- Normal blood pressure is a systolic pressure less than 120 and diastolic pressure less than 80 mm Hg.
- "Prehypertension" is systolic pressure of 120-139 or diastolic pressure of 80-89 mmHg.
- Stage 1 Hypertension is systolic pressure of 140-159 or diastolic pressure of 90-99 mmHg.
- Stage 2 Hypertension is systolic pressure of 160 or greater or diastolic pressure of 100 or greater.
- Stage 3 Hypertension is systolic pressure of 180 or greater or diastolic pressure of 110 or greater

In case of children upto 1 year of age the normal range is systolic 100 to 75 and diastolic 70 to 50. Children from 1 year to upto 5 years of age normal range is systolic 110 to 80 and diastolic 80 to 50. Children from 1 year to upto 3 years of age normal range is systolic 110 to 85 and diastolic blood pressure is 80 to 50. In teenage normal systolic is 120 to 85 and diastolic 80 to 55."

This staging helps doctors to choose the best treatment option for various levels of hypertension.

High blood pressure during pregnancy is a special type of hypertension. If you did not have high blood pressure (diagnosed as hypertensive) before pregnancy, but developed it in the last few months of pregnancy it is hypertension of pregnancy. Usually Blood pressure will return to normal after the baby is born.

Worldwide condition of Hypertension

High blood pressure is a worldwide disease of epidemic proportions. It is a global public health issue. For most doctors, it is the single most common chronic disease encountered in practice. It has been estimated that in Western countries somewhere between 15 and 20 percent of the adult population have high blood pressure.

"A 20-year follow-up study shows that 90% of people gets hypertension in later part of life (age 55 to 85 years)." High blood pressure is relatively rare in children. Among young adults, men are more likely to have it than women. If you are a male over 60 years of age, strong possibility is that you have high blood pressure. But the situation is changing, more young people worldwide are developing hypertension.

"In 2008, approximately 40% of adults aged 25 and above worldwide had been diagnosed with hypertension; the number of people with the condition rose from 600 million in 1980 to 1 billion in 2008. The prevalence of hypertension is highest in the African Region at 46% of adults aged 25 and above, while the lowest prevalence at 35% is found in the USA. Overall, high-income countries have a lower prevalence of hypertension - 35% - than middle or low income country at 40%."

Problems with uncontrolled hypertension

Hypertension or High blood pressure causes many problems when left untreated. It is a major cause of heart disease and stroke. It also causes kidney disease, a specific type of dementia and eye problems. If we do not take steps to control high blood pressure it affects;

Our brain - High blood pressure is one of the leading causes of stroke. As the pressure is high blood vessels supplying brain rupture more often causing stroke. It can also lead to a form of dementia called vascular dementia cause my rupture or destruction of microscopic vessels supplying the brain.

Our heart and blood vessels - High blood pressure can severely damage your blood vessels. Long term uncontrolled hypertension causes enlargement of the heart. Enlargement of heart is dangerous, leading to heart failure.

Our kidneys - kidneys have a very important role in removing waste products from our body. High blood pressure can damage kidneys by damaging its filtering structure and vessels. The interesting thing is, damage to our kidneys also raises blood pressure. This is a dangerous cycle. When uncontrolled this leads to complete failure of kidneys.

Our eyes and limbs - High blood pressure does not just affect internal organs. It also damages the blood vessels throughout the body such as eyes and limbs, causing loss or decreased sight and mobility problems.

Studies show your risk for stroke or heart attack double with only 10 mm Hg rise in blood pressure. So even a small rise is dangerous.

Every year complications of hypertension such as stroke or heart attack or failure is responsible for more than 9.4 million deaths worldwide. Individually Hypertension causes half of the deaths

(51%) due to stroke and almost half (45%) the death due to heart failure.

So, it is crucial that you control your high blood pressure and keep it controlled lifelong for a healthy and long life.

Cause of High Blood Pressure

For most adults, there's no identifiable cause of high blood pressure. Your Blood pressure may gradually rise over the years. This type of high blood pressure, without any specific cause is called primary or essential hypertension. Don't let the name confuse you, the name doesn't mean this blood pressure is primary and needs no control, nor it is essential to keep it high.

On the other hand, some high blood pressure has an underlying identifiable condition or cause. This type of high blood pressure, called secondary hypertension. Because its secondary to a specific cause. Usually secondary hypertension tends to appear suddenly and usually show higher blood pressure level than primary hypertension. We can get secondary Hypertension in following conditions

- Kidney problems
- Adrenal gland tumors
- Thyroid problems
- Certain defects in blood vessels we're born with (congenital)
- Certain medications, such as cold remedies, decongestants, over-the-counter pain relievers and some prescription drugs.
- Illegal drugs, such as cocaine and amphetamines
- Alcohol abuse or chronic alcohol use

Types of Hypertension

As you have read earlier, there are mainly two major types of hypertension

1. Essential hypertension: Essential or the primary hypertension is more common About 90% to 95% of people with hypertension have primary hypertension. This high blood pressure has no identifiable cause. Essential hypertension is diagnosed incidentally after your doctor notices that your blood pressure is higher on three or more visits. Your doctor then looks for and eliminates all causes of hypertension.

Usually people with essential hypertension have no symptoms, but you may experience frequent headaches, tiredness, dizziness, or nose bleeds. Although the cause of essential hypertension is unknown. But obesity, smoking, alcohol, diet, and family history all play a role in this. It is also called Primary Hypertension.

2. Secondary hypertension: In a small percentage of hypertensive patients (about 10%) have an identifiable cause for the condition. It may be caused by another disease. The most common cause of secondary hypertension is an abnormality in the arteries supplying blood to the kidneys. Other causes include airway obstruction during sleep, diseases and tumors of the adrenal glands, hormone abnormalities, thyroid disease, and too much salt or alcohol in the diet. Some drugs can cause secondary hypertension, including over-the-counter medications.

There are some Additional Hypertension Types:

Isolated systolic hypertension: This type of hypertension is more common in people over the age of 65 and is caused by the loss of elasticity of arteries. In isolated systolic hypertension, systolic pressure becomes high, but diastolic pressure is in normal range. For example, a systolic pressure of 140 or greater with a diastolic reading of 89 or below can be called isolated systolic hypertension. This is the most common form of high blood pressure in the elderly.

"The Framingham Heart Study, which has tracked the health of participants since the late 1940s, found that 65% to 75% of people over age 65 with elevated blood pressure had isolated systolic hypertension."

Malignant Hypertension: This type of hypertension occurs in only about 1 percent of people with hypertension. It is more common in younger adults, African-American men, and women who have pregnancy toxemia (a complication of pregnancy). With malignant hypertension, blood pressure rises suddenly and go for a very high level typically above 180/120, sometimes diastolic pressure can go over 130.

Malignant Hypertension is a medical emergency and should be treated immediately in a hospital.

Resistant hypertension: sometimes to control your blood pressure you may need two or more drugs. If your doctor has prescribed three different types of antihypertensive medications together and your blood pressure is still high, then you have resistant hypertension. By definition "Hypertension is called resistant if three medications fail to successfully treat the condition."

At least four medications may be necessary to treat resistant hypertension. This dangerous condition occurs in 20 to 30 percent of hypertensive patients. Resistant hypertension usually has a genetic component and is more common in people who are older, obese, female, African American, or have another illness, such as diabetes or kidney disease.

Renal hypertension: also, called renovascular hypertension. As the name suggests this high blood pressure occurs due to kidney disease. Renal hypertension can usually be controlled by blood pressure drugs.   Sometimes Renal hypertension may need angioplasty, stenting, or surgery on the blood vessels of the kidney. Surgery may cure the condition.

White Coat Hypertension: If high blood pressure occurs only when blood pressure is taken in a clinical setting. And outside of a doctor's office blood pressure is normal. It is called White Coat Hypertension. Patients with white coat hypertension is believed to get extremely stressed when visiting a clinic or doctor's office, causing the blood pressure to shoot up. If you have high blood pressure during a doctor's visit, you should check your blood pressure in other locations such as your home to rule out white coat hypertension.

Sudden High blood pressure: is a specific high blood pressure where there is a sudden and isolated high blood pressure occur. It is usually caused by some practices and habits in our daily life. Some of these are:

Medication use. Overuse of certain drugs can suddenly increase your blood pressure. For example, NSAIDS commonly used as over the counter pain medication such as ibuprofen and aspirin may suddenly raise your blood pressure. Birth control pills and several other drugs when taken together can also cause increased blood pressure suddenly and unexpectedly. Drug abuse with cocaine and marijuana may cause a high in blood pressure unexpectedly.

Smoking. Smoking is dangerous, no doubt about it. There are many chemicals in smoke including nicotine, damage our blood vessels. They also decrease the elasticity of blood vessels, making them unable to cope with higher blood pressure. This can lead to stroke or heart condition. Smoking also causes a sudden increase in blood pressure.

Diet. Bad dietary habits are eating high saturated fat contents and high sodium which is likely to lead to multiple episodes of high blood pressure.

<u>Anxiety and stress</u>. Stress is caused by everyday activities or certain thoughts. Stress affects us on multiple levels. It is a fact that psychological issues such as phobias and depression can cause an unexplained increase in blood pressure, and if such symptoms continue, then it increases the risk of developing hypertension.

<u>Other causes</u>. Overuse of stimulating drinks such as tea, coffee, energy drinks and alcohol can cause a sudden increase in the blood pressure for a short period. Increased weight, pain and hormonal imbalance can also cause a sudden increase in the blood pressure. In some cases, pregnancy can lead to sudden high blood pressure.

Symptoms of Hypertension

Usually the only way we find out that we have high blood pressure when it is measured. It is alarming to know that more than 68 million Americans have hypertension and 33% of them doesn't even know it. The disease is increasingly affecting more and more by almost 15 to 18 million or more every 10 years.

Most of the time there is no symptom of Hypertension. You may have a common misconception that people with hypertension always experience symptoms, but the reality is most hypertensive people have no symptoms at all. Over time severe damage to your arteries, heart, and brain can occur before hypertension is diagnosed. That's why Hypertension is called "Silent killer".

Hypertension is usually diagnosed by a health care professional during a routine checkup.

Sometimes and not in everyone hypertension causes symptoms such as headache, shortness of breath, dizziness, chest pain, palpitations and nose bleeds. If you have any of these symptoms Do not ignore them, but these symptoms do not confirm that you have hypertension. You may have these symptoms for other diseases. It is always wise to report symptoms to your doctor as well as to have your blood pressure regularly checked. If you have risk factors such as obesity, smoking, high cholesterol and family history of hypertension, it is especially important to pay attention to your blood pressure reading. Increasing age more than 55 years also needs regular blood pressure monitoring at least every 6 months.

Sometimes when blood pressure becomes extremely high, you may have unusually strong headache, chest pain, difficulty breathing, or difficulty breathing during physical work or exercise. If you have any of these symptoms, consult your doctor for an evaluation as soon as possible.

Risk factors for developing high blood pressure

Family history

We inherit risk of hypertension just as we inherit hair and eye color. If your parents or close blood relatives have had hypertension, you are more likely to develop it. You might also pass this risk factor on to your children. So, it's important for children as well as adults to have regular blood pressure checks if family history of hypertension is positive.

You can't control the risk factor you inherit, but you can take steps to prevent hypertension and live a healthy life. You can easily lower your other risk factors. Through Lifestyle choices you can prevent hypertension even if you have a strong family history of hypertension.

Race/Ethnicity

"High blood pressure is more common in African American adults than in Caucasian or Hispanic American adults. Compared to other ethnic groups, African Americans Tend to get high blood pressure earlier in life. On average African Americans have higher blood pressure numbers. You have to double your efforts to control hypertension if you are an African American".

Advanced age

The alarming reality is that most of us will get high blood pressure when we are 60 or more. As we age, we all develop a higher risk for high blood pressure and cardiovascular disease. With ageing blood vessels lose flexibility and become hard. This causes increased blood pressure. The chance of rupture of blood vessels causing stroke or heart attack.

Gender-related risk patterns

Gender plays a mixed pattern in case of high blood pressure. Upto 45 years' women get hypertension more than men, then in the age group 45 to 64 both men and women gets it in similar rate then again after age 64 the chance is more in women in getting high blood pressure. So, women should be extra cautious about high blood pressure.

Lack of physical activity

Physical activity is good for your heart and circulatory system. A physically inactive lifestyle increases chance of high blood pressure, heart disease, blood vessel disease and stroke. Inactivity also makes it easier to become overweight or obese. Obesity also is a strong risk factor of high blood pressure.

Diet

Diet plays a major role in causing or preventing high blood pressure. Now almost everyone knows that a diet high in salt and fat and low in nutritional value increased risk for High Blood Pressure. The point is to apply this to our life. We all need good nutrition from a variety of food sources. A diet that's high in calories, fats and sugars and low in essential nutrients also lead to unhealthy heart as well as to obesity leading to hypertension.

In addition, salt is another important factor. Some people are "salt sensitive," meaning a high-salt (sodium) diet raises their high blood pressure. Salt keeps excess fluid in the body causing increased blood volume. With increased blood volume, your heart has to work more with more force causing rise in blood pressure.

On the other side, healthy food choices can actually lower blood pressure and prevent it.

Overweight and obesity

Being overweight increases your chances of developing high blood pressure. A body mass index between 25 and 30 is considered overweight. A body mass index over 30 is considered obese.

Excess weight increases the strain on the heart, raises blood cholesterol and triglyceride levels, and lowers HDL (good) cholesterol levels. If you lose as little as 10 to 20 pounds it can help lower your blood pressure and that's a start.

You can easily calculate your body mass index using web apps available online. If the weight is not in ideal range you need to manage your weight.

Alcohol

Heavy and regular use of alcohol can increase blood pressure dramatically. It can also cause heart failure, stroke and irregular heartbeats. If you drink, limit your alcohol consumption to no more than two drinks per day for men and one drink per day for women.

Other Possible contributing factors for developing high blood pressure

There is some connection between blood pressure and the following factors but study has not proven yet that they actually cause high blood pressure.

Stress

We have a common conception that stress and stressful situation causes high blood pressure. Stress and stressful condition temporarily increase blood pressure, but study has not proven that stress can cause long term high blood pressure. Some studies show a relationship between coronary heart disease risk and stress in a person's life. Some people under stress eats more and eats less healthy diet to cope with stressful situations. They may put off physical activity, drink, smoke or misuse drugs. All these results in increased risk of developing hypertension.

Smoking and second-hand smoke

There is no excuse of smoking. You need to stop, make others stop smoking. Smoking temporarily raises blood pressure causing damaged arteries. So even a single stick is harmful. Secondhand smoke or exposure to other people's smoke increases the risk of heart disease in nonsmokers. You should kick the habit as soon as you can.

The new trend of Vape is still too new to comment. The nicotine in vape is known to rise blood pressure temporarily. Vape needs long term study to be declared safe or unsafe.

Sleep Apnea

"Some 12 million Americans have sleep apnea", according to National Heart, Lung, and Blood Institute. Sleep Apnea is a unusual but now common sleep disorder in which tissues in the throat collapse and block the airway during sleep. Then brain forces the sleeper awake enough to cough or gulp air and open the trachea. But after a few minutes, the whole cycle starts all over again. This inadequate sleep for a long time causes severe fatigue during the day make it difficult to perform tasks that require alertness. Sleep apnea is a proven risk factor for high blood pressure, heart failure, diabetes and stroke. Obesity may play a major role in sleep apnea.

Diagnosis of Hypertension

Hypertension does not show any obvious symptom unless there are complications such as stroke, heart failure, kidney disease etc. Hypertension is usually diagnosed by a health care professional during a routine checkup.

Blood pressure levels are not as stable as cholesterol or body weight, but tend to vary in every measurement. Usually during the first visit to the doctor's office blood pressure reading is higher. Also, blood pressure is usually higher in first measurement than if its measured 2 or 3 times 10 minutes apart. Good thing this false high blood pressure tends to become normal in following visits.

So, you can't be diagnosed as hypertensive in one isolated visit. Usually repeated measurements taken during at least 2 to 3 different visits to the doctor's office is needed to confirm the diagnosis of Hypertension.

The diagnosis of hypertension is made when either the systolic blood pressure is persistently higher than 140 mmHg or when the diastolic is higher than 90 mmHg or two conditions coexist.

Sometimes we need to monitor blood pressure for 24 hours before we can be certain about the diagnosis of hypertension.

Steps for Blood Pressure Measurement

Usually blood pressure is monitored manually with a mercury column or mechanical aneroid sphygmomanometer. Now automated BP devices are also used and recommended. American Heart Association (AHA) states "there is a role for (automated) devices in office use, both as a substitute for traditional (manual) readings and as supplements to them."

It does not matter if you use an automatic monitor or a manual one, you need to follow some guideline to measure blood pressure accurately.

Need right equipment:

- For manual measurement, you will need a quality stethoscope. In automated device, you don't need stethoscope.
- An appropriately sized blood pressure cuff. Most measurement errors occur due to inappropriate cuff size. The cuff should encircle at least 80% of the circumference and cover two thirds of the length of the arm. Wrap the cuff around the arm and use the INDEX line to determine if arm circumference falls within the RANGE area. Otherwise, choose the smaller or larger cuff.
- A larger or smaller cuff than your actual size will give incorrect results. Your doctor or health care professional will help to choose the right cuff size for you.
- You can use manual blood pressure measurement instrument or an automated device with a manual inflate mode.

Preparation:

- You need to relax at least 5 minutes before taking first reading.
- It's best to remove excess clothing that might interfere with the cuff placement or tighten blood flow in the arm.
- Sit upright in a chair with upper arm positioned at the level with heart and feet flat on the floor.
- Don't talk during measurement.

Placement of the BP cuff:

- Locate the brachial artery and position the BP cuff so that the ARTERY marker points to the brachial artery. Wrap the BP cuff snugly around the arm.

Position the stethoscope:

- If you are measuring blood pressure manually then on the same arm that you wrapped cuff place the bell of the stethoscope over the crease of the arm called antecubical fossa here an artery called brachial artery is located.

Inflate the BP cuff:

- Begin pumping the cuff bulb. When manually measuring the BP, you need to inflate the cuff enough to stop blood flow. When blood flow stops, you should hear no sounds through the stethoscope. Generally, you can inflate the cuff to 160 - 180 mmHg. When measuring using an automatic device follow the instruction given with the device.

Slowly Deflate the BP cuff:

- If measuring manually begin deflation of the cuff slowly. The AHA recommends "the pressure should fall 2 - 3 mmHg per second, anything faster may likely result in an inaccurate measurement". In automatic device follow the instruction.

Listen for the Systolic Reading:

- Listen with the stethoscope while deflating the cuff slowly. The first occurrence of rhythmic sounds resembling a tapping noise heard as blood begins to flow through the artery. Note the gauge reading when the tapping sound starts. This is the systolic pressure.

Listen for the Diastolic Reading:

- Continue to listen while deflating cuff. As the cuff pressure drops the sounds slowly fades. Note the gauge reading when the rhythmic sounds fade. This is the diastolic reading.

Check Again:

- The AHA recommends "taking a reading with both arms and averaging the readings." You need to check the pressure again, wait about five minutes between readings. Take two readings on each arm and average the reading for maximum accuracy.

Incorrect blood pressure measurement

Some factors affect blood pressure measurement when you are measuring it manually. You can get an incorrect reading such as too high or too low with faulty technique. Following are some tips to help you with correct measurements.

- Inflating the cuff too slowly or not inflating it to a high enough pressure may cause a false reading. If you loosen the valve too much and deflate the cuff too quickly, you will not be able to measure your blood pressure.
- It is normal for your blood pressure to vary at different times of the day: It is usually higher when you are at work. It drops slightly at home. Blood pressure is usually lower when sleeping. It is normal for your blood pressure to increase suddenly when you wake up.
- Blood pressure readings taken at home are a better measure of your blood pressure than those taken at doctor's office. This is called white coat hypertension, in some people it causes unusually high blood pressure at doctor's office.
- Blood pressure readings can be influenced by factors like: Smoking, Coffee or other caffeinated drinks, A full bladder,

Recent physical activity or stress. Try avoiding them before measuring.

- Posture during measure - if you are 65 or more years old, with diabetes and taking antihypertensive therapy you should check your blood pressure in 2 position. Measure lying flat on bed then again in standing position. It shows if there is a major drop in BP when you are standing, it may cause blackout or loss of consciousness and needs consultation with your doctor.

Since so many factors can influence blood pressure readings, you should have your blood pressure taken several times 5 to 10 minutes apart to get an accurate measurement. The recommended guideline is using a 7-day measurement period with two to three measurements each morning and two to three measurements in the evening. Exclude the first-day measurements from the analyses to remove the alerting reaction. Calculate an average of 12 morning and 12 evening measurements.

This calculated average is your true Blood pressure.

24 hours Ambulatory blood pressure measurement (ABPM)

Sometimes we need to check blood pressure for 24 hours to confirm the diagnosis of hypertension. The 24 hours monitoring of blood pressure is also called Ambulatory blood pressure (ABP) monitoring. The procedure automatically measures blood pressure at regular intervals (every 20–30 minutes) using an automatic device over a 24-hour period while you undergo normal daily activities and sleep.

ABPM device is a small digital blood pressure monitoring device that is attached to a belt around your body. It has a cuff which is wrapped around your upper arm. The device is small and you can and need to do your normal daily activity and even sleep with it on to get the correct measurement.

ABPM checks your blood pressure automatically every 20 to 30 min for 24 hours. Before starting the measurement, it gives a beeping sound.

When 24 hours are complete, the data from the device collected. A trained professional analyzes the data to give a complete picture of your blood pressure changes throughout the day with an average systolic and diastolic BP and heart rate.

ABPM is useful;

- To confirm the diagnosis of hypertension ABPM is the best option.
- To rule out white coat hypertension. Using ABPM, we can find out if the high blood pressure readings in the clinic are higher than they are away from the clinic.
- To see how medicines are working to control your blood pressure.
- To adjust the dose of medicine and make sure medicines are controlling blood pressure throughout the day.
- If there is a need to change or adjust medicines.

The National Institute for Health and Care Excellence (NICE) guideline recommends that "if a clinic blood pressure is 140/90 mm Hg or higher, ABPM should be offered to confirm the diagnosis of hypertension". Ambulatory blood pressure monitoring is needed in the following conditions;

- Drug resistance if your blood pressure is not controlled even with 2 or more drug.

- If there is kidney, liver or heart disease
- Hypertension during pregnancy.
- Patients with associated disease such as diabetes.
- In case of White coat hypertension
- Sudden Fluctuation of BP with change of posture.
- Elderly patients with isolated systolic hypertension."

To allow the 24-hour monitoring machine to work properly, it is important to make sure that the tube to the machine from cuff is not twisted, blocked or bent. Just before the machine is about to take a reading, it will beep. When it beeps, you should:

- Sit down, if possible
- Keep the cuff at the same level as your heart
- Keep your arm steady.

Choosing a device to measure Hypertension at home

Your treatment, dose adjustment and lifestyle modification depend on the blood pressure levels. The more data you have the best are the chance of treatment. It's best to get a home blood pressure monitor and check blood pressure at home.

If you decide to measure your blood pressure at home, choosing a home blood pressure monitor is very important. You should choose a monitor which gives accurate result. There are many different kinds of home blood pressure monitor available.

- It is easiest to use a monitor that is fully automatic.
- Choose one that measures your blood pressure at your upper arm. Try not to use monitors that use wrist or finger. Wrist or finger blood pressure monitors may give incorrect

results. Upper-arm blood pressure monitors usually is the most accurate.

- Always choose Blood pressure monitor that has been clinically validated. Make sure the monitor has been tested, validated and approved by any one of the Association for the Advancement of Medical Instrumentation or British Hypertension Society or the International Protocol for the Validation of Automated BP Measuring Devices.

- The device has ha cuff that you have to wrap around your upper arm. Most home blood pressure monitors will come with a medium-sized cuff. Make sure the cuff is right size for you. If you use a cuff that is either large or small for you, your blood pressure reading will not be correct. Children and adults with smaller or larger than average-sized arms may need special-sized cuffs. Take help from your doctor to know the cuff size perfect for you. You may have to order a specific sized cuff separately.

- When selecting a blood pressure monitor for the elderly, pregnant women or children, make sure it can be used for these conditions. Ensure the monitor is programmed for your special needs.

- Choose a digital monitor to suit your budget. Blood pressure monitors can vary in price. This usually depends on the number of extra features it has. Extra features can be helpful but they are not necessary. You may not need many extra features for example a built-in memory. Choose a device that go easy on your wallet.

- All the automatic blood pressure monitors need to be calibrated, usually every two years. For accurate result make sure it's calibrated.

Ask your healthcare professional for advice in selecting and using a device to monitor your blood pressure at home. It's necessary to have the device checked by your healthcare provider when it's new and if possible once a year to make sure the readings are accurate.

How often should you visit your doctor?

Initially after confirming your diagnosis of hypertension, follow up visits to the doctor should be every few weeks, it is due to verify the diagnosis of hypertension. During these visits, your doctor will estimate the cardiovascular risk and choose the appropriate treatment   strategy.

When your blood pressure is well controlled you may visit your doctor every 6 months for evaluation of cardiovascular risk. If there are other associated risk factors present such as high cholesterol, diabetes mellitus, smoking, renal disease, heart disease, stroke or when hypertension is difficult to control you should see your doctor every 2 to 3 months.

Unfortunately, some hypertensive patients give up their treatment or follow up after a certain period of time. This is because they think that if their blood pressure is normal for sometimes they are "cured" and do not need drugs anymore. Sometimes patient experience an adverse reaction to the treatment and avoid follow up. Sometimes patients stop follow up just because they forgot to take their medication or visit their doctor.

This is dangerous because poorly controlled hypertension leads to many risks including stroke, heart attack. If you are followed-up on a regular basis and keep your blood pressure well controlled, these risks can be avoided.

Treatment of hypertension is a lifelong process. We still don't have a cure for the condition. Effective cooperation between you and your doctor is needed to effectively control blood pressure. You need to continue treatment to accomplish of its long-term therapeutic targets.

PART TWO

TREATMENT OPTIONS FOR HIGH BLOOD PRESSURE

Hypertension is a chronic disease, it means you have to be prepared to continue treatment for a long time, sometimes even the rest of your life, even if your high blood pressure becomes normal. But as your diagnosis is confirmed as high blood pressure you face a common confusion. There are many treatment options available. Choosing the right treatment plan is very important, but confusing.

If you know some general information about the treatment options available, you can discuss your thoughts or plans with your doctor. Keep in mind your doctor is the best person to advise your treatment but it's you who will decide the treatment plan. With information, you can take a correct and informed decision.

General Treatment Guideline for High Blood Pressure

Treatment of hypertension depends on multiple factors. Most of the time the treatment to control high blood pressure is individualized. Sometimes you will need to go through some trial and error to choose the medicine and dose right for you. Your doctor plays a significant role in choosing the best treatment.

Following are some treatment guideline used by doctors worldwide to treat hypertension

Prehypertension

American Guidelines for Hypertension (JNC-7, 2003) use the term prehypertension. In prehypertension, the systolic reading is within 120 mmHg to 139 mmHg, or the diastolic reading is within 80 mmHg to 89 mmHg. Both systolic and diastolic can be high.

Prehypertension is a warning sign that you may get high blood pressure in near future. The term prehypertension is used to create early awareness of Hypertension. According to the American Heart Association, "59 million people in the U.S. have prehypertension".

But on the other hand, European Society of Hypertension, British Society of Hypertension and Hellenic Society for The Study of Hypertension do not use the term or classification of Prehypertension.

According to those guidelines systolic pressure between 120 mmHg to 129 mmHg, or the diastolic pressure between 80 mmHg to 84 mmHg is normal range of blood pressure. According to these guidelines Systolic pressure 130 to 139 mmHg or diastolic 85 to 89 mmHg, or both are termed as High normal blood pressure.

People with prehypertension or High normal blood pressure have a greater risk of other cardiovascular disease such as stroke. Most of the time risk factors for hypertension such as high cholesterol, obesity, and diabetes are seen more in people with prehypertension than in those with normal blood pressure.

The goal of Prehypertension is to start lifestyle changes early for the prevention of hypertension. Prehypertension needs monitoring of blood pressure regularly so it allows prompt treatment if blood pressure becomes higher.

Treatment with drugs or medicines is not necessary in prehypertension stage.

Here are some strategies to help you manage prehypertension:

- Lose weight if you are overweight. Overweight people has risk of developing prehypertension 20% more. On the other hand, even modest amount of weight loss reduces the risk.
- Exercise regularly. Exercise helps you lose weight. Exercise also helps lower blood pressure.
- Eat plenty of fruits, vegetables, whole grains, fish, and low-fat dairy. A specific diet plan such as DASH can prevent hypertension as well as lower blood pressure.

- Reduce salt/sodium in your diet. You should take less than 2,300 milligrams of sodium per day (2300mg is about 1 teaspoon of table salt).

It's important to get your blood pressure checked regularly. You can monitor your blood pressure between doctor's visits with a home blood pressure monitor.

Stage 1 Hypertension

If your systolic blood pressure is between 140 and 159 or your diastolic pressure between 90 and 99, you are considered to be in hypertension stage 1. Stage 1 hypertension occurs more frequently in older individuals (age 65 and more), women and African Americans.

Untreated stage 1 hypertension leads to atherosclerosis. In atherosclerosis arteries become hard and lost its elasticity with increased risk of stroke, heart attack and kidney disease. In stage 1 hypertension your heart needs to work harder to pump the blood inside the body.

At stage 1 hypertension start with lifestyle modification, there is a strong possibility that you will not need any drugs to control stage 1 hypertension. But some of us will need to take medicine to control blood pressure even on stage 1. The JNC 7 report recommends that "the first medication to use is a thiazide-type diuretic". A diuretic is a medication that lowers blood pressure by helping your body get rid of extra fluid. Diuretics are usually very effective, have fewer side effects, and are inexpensive. Diuretics are used not only to reduce blood pressure but also to reduce the risk of heart disease and stroke.

If you are African-American risk for complications of hypertension is higher. So the current guideline is that African Americans with blood pressure 145mm Hg or more should start with a combined blood pressure medicine.

Stage 2 Hypertension

According to current guidelines Systolic blood pressure is 160 mm Hg or higher or diastolic 100 mm Hg or higher is called stage 2 hypertension. Stage 2 hypertension is also known as late high blood pressure or severe high blood pressure.

Stage 2 hypertension is a serious form of high blood pressure. It needs more frequent blood pressure checks and more careful monitoring.

If you have Stage 2 Hypertension you must consult your doctor and start immediate treatment. Initially you have to start lifestyle changes, including:

- Quit smoking.
- Maintain a healthy weight.
- Consume a diet rich in fruits, vegetables and low-fat dairy products.
- Limit salt in your diet.
- Limit alcohol intake.
- Exercise at least 30 minutes per day. Simple aerobic exercise such as walking, jogging, strength training, yoga or cardio workout like cycling.

In stage 2 hypertension it's a strong possibility that In addition to lifestyle changes you will need medicine preferably a two-drug therapy. It will be advised by your doctor. Following drugs are usually used to treat Stage 2 hypertension:

- ACE inhibitors – they allow blood vessels to widen by preventing angiotensin (a hormone) from forming.

- Angiotensin II receptor blockers - by blocking the action of angiotensin these drugs allow blood vessels to relax.
- Beta blockers - block specific nerve and hormone signals to your heart and blood vessels causing relaxed heart and blood vessel leading to lower blood pressure.
- Calcium channel blockers - prevent calcium ions from going into heart mussels and blood vessel muscle causing a widening of blood vessels leading to lower blood pressure.
- Renin inhibitors - slow down the production of renin, which is an enzyme produced by your kidneys that increases blood pressure. Without renin, your blood pressure lowers to a normal level.

Stage 3 Hypertension

Stage 3 is an extremely high blood pressure. In stage 3 pressure becomes more than 180/110 mmHg. It is also called sever hypertension. Stage 3 hypertension needs urgent medical treatment with close monitoring.

Remember, stage 3 hypertension is a medical emergency and may need treatment in a hospital setting.

Lifestyle Modification to control hypertension

Every drug has some side effect so initially you should start with lifestyle modification. Life style modification can control your blood pressure dramatically without any medicine. As it is the Natural way to control blood pressure it is best for you in ling term. There are lots of studies to prove that lifestyle modification can control and even prevent high blood pressure.

By lifestyle modification we grossly mean modification of your diet, some exercise, stop smoking and limiting your alcoholic beverages. There is a strong possibility that you wouldn't need to take any medicine to keep high blood pressure in control if you properly modify your lifestyle.

Modify your Diet

Diet is used as a treatment in high blood pressure. Modification of your diet may control your blood pressure without any medicine. On the other hand, you may be at an increased risk for getting high blood pressure if you eat a diet that's low on fiber, high in fat and salt, drink alcohol to excess and smoke.

A good diet not only help controlling high blood pressure, it can also prevent it.

- As a general rule, you should eat plenty of
    - Fruits
    - Vegetables
    - Whole grains
    - Fish
    - Low-fat dairy
    - Low in sodium
- Your diet should be
    - High in potassium

- o Magnesium
- o Calcium
- o Protein
- o Fiber.
- Avoid foods high in saturated fat such as meats and high-fat dairy. Control trans fat such some margarine, snack foods, and pastries in your diet. Limit high cholesterol containing foods such as organ meats, high-fat dairy, and egg yolks. Eat foods low in saturated and trans-fat and cholesterol, read food labels to choose.
- Eat plant based or vegetarian diet at least 2 days every week. You can add high-protein soy foods to your diet. Increase fruits and vegetables.
- Salt keeps excess fluid in the body causing heart to work more. That is a burden on the heart. You must limit salt in your diet. Studies have proven that "A low-sodium diet can lower high blood pressure". According to recommendation you should aim for less than 2,300 milligrams of sodium (salt) daily which is about 1 teaspoon of table salt.
- Drinking excess alcohol increase blood pressure. Limit drinking.

DASH Diet

The DASH diet is a specific diet for patients of High Blood Pressure. It is proven in many studies and highly recommended to control your blood pressure. If you don't want to take medicine for your high blood pressure and plan to control it naturally then this specific diet is the answer.

 DASH stands for Dietary Approaches to Stop Hypertension. In research studies, people who were on the DASH diet lowered their blood pressure within 2 weeks. Some extensive studies found the following health benefits of the DASH diet.

"DASH (Dietary Approaches to Stop Hypertension Trial): This trial included 459 adults, some with and without diagnosed high blood pressure, and compared three diets including 3,000 mg daily sodium.

- Result - Participants on the DASH diet had the greatest effect of lowering their high blood pressure. The DASH diet lowers blood pressure and LDL (bad) cholesterol compared with a typical American diet alone or a typical American diet with more fruits and vegetables.

DASH-Sodium (DASH Diet, Sodium Intake, and Blood Pressure Trial): This trial randomly assigned 412 participants to a typical American diet or the DASH diet. While on their assigned diet, participants were followed for a month at a high daily sodium level (3,300 mg) and two lower daily sodium levels (2,300 mg and 1,500 mg).

- Result - Blood pressure decreased with each reduction of sodium. The DASH Sodium diet lowers blood pressure better than a typical American diet at three daily sodium levels. Combining the DASH diet with sodium reduction gives greater health benefits than the DASH diet alone.

The PREMIER clinical trial: The PREMIER trial included 810 participants who were placed into three groups to lower blood pressure, lose weight, and improve health. After 6 months, blood pressure levels declined in all three groups.

- Result - Participants in the established treatment plan who followed the DASH diet had the greatest improvement in their blood pressure. People can lose weight and lower their blood pressure by following the DASH eating plan and increasing their physical activity".

The DASH diet is simple:

- Eat more fruits, vegetables, and low-fat dairy foods

- Avoid foods that are high in saturated fat, cholesterol, and trans fats
- Eat more whole-grain foods, fish, poultry, and nuts
- Limit sodium, sweets, sugary drinks, and red meats

DASH-Sodium – is a modified DASH diet cutting back salt (sodium) to 1,500 milligrams a day. 1500 mg salt is about two third (2/3) of a teaspoon. This amount includes all sodium taken per day. Including sodium in food products, used in cooking and taken at the table.

Starting DASH diet

The DASH diet is based on certain number of servings daily from various food groups. Depending on the calorie requirement the number of serving is estimated. It is individualized and usually calculated by a dietitian. But you may calculate your calorie need. And adjusts your diet according to DASH plan.

The DASH diet is calculated with serving. When you're trying to follow DASH diet, you need to know the volume of a certain kind of food is considered a "serving." One serving is:

- 1/2 cup cooked rice or pasta is considered a "serving."
- 1 slice bread is considered a "serving."
- 1 cup raw vegetables or fruit is considered a "serving."
- 1/2 cup cooked veggies or fruit is considered a "serving."
- 8 ounces of milk is considered a "serving."
- 1 teaspoon of olive oil (or any other oil) is considered a "serving."
- 3 ounces of cooked meat is considered a "serving."
- 3 ounces of tofu is considered a "serving."

Following is a sample daily and weekly DASH Eating Plan to give you an idea of the diet. This sample plan sets goal for a 2,000 Calorie per day:

- Grains: 7-8 servings daily
- Vegetables: 4-5 servings daily
- Fruits: 4-5 servings daily
- Fat free or Low fat dairy products: 2-3 servings daily
- Meat, poultry, and fish: less than 2 daily servings
- Nuts, seeds, and dry beans: weekly 4-5 servings
- Fats and oils: less than 3 servings daily
- Sweets: try to limit to less than 5 servings per week.

You need specific changes in the DASH diet if you have other associated conditions such as Diabetes or high cholesterol.

For DASH Sodium diet - You can limit your salt intake gradually. Start by limiting to 2,400 milligrams of salt (sodium) per day. It's about 1 teaspoon of table salt. Then, once you have adjusted to the low salt diet, cut back to 1,500 milligrams of salt (sodium) per day which is about 2/3 of a teaspoon. These amounts include all sodium eaten, including sodium in food products as well as in what you cook with or add at the table.

Tips on DASH diet

Following are some tips you can use when on DASH or DASH Sodium diet:

- Always add a serving of vegetables at lunch and at dinner.
- Add a serving of fruit to your meals or as a snack. Canned and dried fruits are easy to use, but make sure by reading the label that they don't have added sugar or salt.
- Use low-fat or fat free and only half your typical serving of butter, margarine, or salad dressing.
- Drink low-fat or skim dairy products instead of full fat or full cream.

- Limit meat to 6 ounces a day. Make some meals vegetarian.
- Add more vegetables and beans to your diet.
- Unsalted pretzels or nuts, raisins, low-fat or fat-free yogurt, unsalted popcorn without butter or oil, and raw vegetables is good snaking choice.
- You should always read food labels to choose products that are low in salt and fat.

Every individual is different. Our food choices are different so you should consult a dietitian to get a specific DASH diet plan tailored according to your need and food habit.

Pritikin Diet

There is another Popular diet plan available for high blood pressure called Pritikin diet. The Pritikin Principle or diet is a low-fat diet based on vegetables, grains, and fruits. Nathan Pritikin invented the plan. Robert Pritikin improved the diet. Plant-based foods with very low fat are mainly used in Pritikin diet. The latest Pritikin diet focuses on a latest concept called calorie density solution.

With calorie density, the concern is not calories in various food but rather how dense they are in any given food. The idea is to choose foods that are not "calorie dense," meaning they have relatively low calories per pound. For example, a pound of raw broccoli has 130 calories (without butter) and a pound of chocolate chip cookies has 2,140 calories.

How the Pritikin Principle Works

Pritikin diet suggests we eat whole, unprocessed, and natural carbohydrate rich foods, such as grains, vegetables, and fruit. Preferred foods include:

- Brown rice
- Millet
- Barley
- Oats
- Dark green, leafy vegetables
- Onions
- Potatoes
- Squash
- Beans (black turtle beans, chickpeas, lentils, lima and pinto beans)
- Apples
- Pears
- Strawberries
- Bananas

Some processed whole-grain foods, such as oatmeal, white-flour pasta can be included in your diet, as long as you eat it with vegetables.

Other guidelines in Pritikin diet are:

- You can eat small servings of lean beef, chicken, and low-fat dairy products.
- Including fish in your diet is encouraged. Pritikin diet suggest at least three servings of fish per week of salmon or other fish rich in omega-3 fatty acids.
- You have to avoid fried foods, dressing with fat, and fatty sauces.
- Eat three meals a day plus two snacks.
- Avoid salty foods.
- Artificial sweeteners can be used in Pritikin diet.

The Pritikin program gives dramatic results. Blood pressure start to falls quickly. Studies on the Pritikin Program have shown that this diet reduces the need of blood pressure medicine in many people.

One study with 1117 high blood pressure patients shown that on average with Pritikin diet blood pressure is reduced 9% or more. 45% of the patients lowered their high blood pressure medicine and stunning 55% stopped high blood pressure medicine achieving normal range of blood pressure.

You can choose to try both diets (DASH or PRITIKIN) alternatively to see which one works better for you.

Exercise

Due to urban life and development of technology such as (TV, Computer and mobiles) we have developed a physically inactive lifestyle. Most of our time is spent in sitting or lying using computer, games or mobile, even in the office. This leads to risk factors. Physical inactivity is a major risk factor for developing high blood pressure and the risk increases with age.

Exercise can make a big difference in the prevention of hypertension. And if your blood pressure is already high, exercise can help you control it. Scientific studies have shown that "regular exercise reduces blood pressure by an average of 6-7 mmHg". That's as good as some blood pressure medications.

For some of hypertensive patients, exercise is enough to reduce blood pressure. There is no need of any blood pressure medication. During exercise your blood pressure may become a bit high but the pressure becomes low afterwards. Studies have shown the effect of only 30 minutes of exercise has an immediate blood pressure lowering effect lasting minutes to hours.

What Type of Exercise Is Best for Hypertension

There are three basic types of exercise:

- Easy aerobic exercise such as walking, jogging, jumping rope, bicycling (stationary or outdoor), cross-country skiing, skating, rowing, high- or low-impact aerobics and swimming. Aerobic exercise works best in lowering your blood pressure and make your heart stronger.
- Walking is one of the most effective exercise for all levels of high blood pressure and for every age group. Walking gives the best result.

- Strength training builds strong muscles that help you burn more calories throughout the day. It's also good for your joints and bones.
- Stretching makes you more flexible, helps you move better, and helps prevent injury.

So how does exercise work? Regular physical activity or exercise makes your heart stronger. A stronger heart can pump more blood with less effort. If your heart can work less (low heart beat) to pump, the force on your arteries decreases, lowering your blood pressure. Also during exercise there is a temporary increase in your heart rate along with blood pressure, it has a cleansing effect on your blood vessels removing plaques blocking it.

The exact duration and type of exercise for blood pressure management is not important. However, the current guidelines listed by the American College of Sports Medicine recommend "you should start with 30 minutes of moderate aerobic exercise in the form of walking, running or cycling at least five days per week. Regular physical activity at least 30 minutes most days of the week can lower your blood pressure by 4 to 9 millimeters of mercury (mm Hg). Remember that you need to be consistent in your workout, if you stop regular exercising, your blood pressure becomes high again.

Research has found that too much sedentary time can contribute to many health conditions including high blood pressure. If in your workplace, you have to sit for long hours every day, try to break the amount of time as hourly chunks. Do any physical activity for 5 minutes, you may get up to get a drink of water or walk a little inside the office or climb some stairs every hour. Consider setting a reminder in your to do list, calendar or on your smartphone. Following are some tips to help you;

- Exercise at the same time every day. It will become a regular part of your routine, and it will be harder to skip.
- Wear comfortable clothes when you work out.
- It's best to take your blood pressure before and after you exercise.
- Set realistic goals for yourself that you think you can achieve.
- Find an exercise "buddy." This will help you stay motivated and enjoy it more.

Most people with high blood pressure can exercise safely. But as exercise makes your heart work harder, you need to be careful, especially if you're just starting or your blood pressure is moderately or very high. If your blood pressure is moderately high (stage 2 hypertension), you may need to take medicine to reach a lower level of blood pressure before you may start exercising. If your blood pressure is very high (stage 3 hypertension), you should not start any new activity without consulting your doctor. In general;

- If your Blood pressure level is below 90/60 or lower then you have low blood pressure, It may lead to dizziness even fainting, speak to your doctor or nurse before starting any new exercise with low blood pressure.
- If Blood pressure in the range of 90/60-140/90 It is safe to exercise and be more active.
- If your Blood pressure in range of 140/90 – 179/99. It is safe to exercise with moderate intensity.
- If Blood pressure in range of 180/100 – 199/109. You should consult your doctor before starting any kind of exercise.
- If Blood pressure in range of 200/110 or above. Do not start any exercise without consulting your doctor first. You have

to take medicine to lower your blood pressure before you can take any kind of exercise.

Specific tips on Exercise with Hypertension.

To keep up healthy heart and control high blood pressure you don't need vigorous exercise. Easy aerobic exercise is enough. Studies show simple exercise such as aerobic exercise if done regularly reduce blood pressure 10 points or more.

Avoid competitive or high intensity exercises that include bursts of intense exertion. Avoid weights for exercise or use it carefully. Resistance training can lower blood pressure by 2 to 4 percent, but if your blood pressure is 160/100 or more, you should not lift weights. Only if your doctor approves lifting weights you may do it. If you have your doctor's approval, do one set of 10 to 15 reps using a moderate weight. Try not to hold your breath while lifting, try to exhale when lifting or exerting effort.

After stretching or exercising on the floor, get up slowly. Some blood pressure medications can make you dizzy or sometimes complete black out when you stand or getup quickly. It is called "Orthostatic Hypotension,". It occurs when blood pressure suddenly drops to a very low pressure with a sudden change of posture.

Skip Caffeine before exercise. A cup of coffee before workout may cause a sudden high in your blood pressure. It is best to avoid caffeine 3 to 4 hours before exercising.

And when working out, remember: always warm up first and cool down after finishing by stretching. This will help your heart to slowly adjust to the activity.

Making exercise a habit can help you continue with the routine. Exercise gives you more energy, and it's a great way to ease stress and feel better. Start by brisk walking, jogging, swimming, biking or doing yard work.

How Often Should You Exercise

Usually it is best to do a moderate exercise such as walking. Walk for 30 min everyday or at least walk 5 days weekly. If you choose more active workout such as jogging, swimming you can work out for 20 minutes at least 5 days. It has the same benefit as 30 min walking.

You can start slow and gradually increase the time. When starting an exercise, warm up for 5 to 10 minutes first to increase your heart rate slowly. Warming up also helps prevent injury. Then, step up the intensity.

When finishing it's best not to stop suddenly. This is especially important if you have high blood pressure. Just slow down for a few minutes. This gives your body a chance to cool down.

When you should stop exercising

If you are starting an exercise with hypertension for the first time It may take a while before your body gets used to exercise. It is normal to breathe harder and to sweat, it's normal for your heart to beat faster when you're doing exercise.

But if you're feeling very short of breath, or difficulty in breathing or if you feel like your heart is beating too fast or irregularly, stop exercising and rest.

Stop exercising if you feel chest pain, weakness, dizziness, lightheadedness, or pressure or pain in your neck, left arm, left jaw, or left shoulder. If these symptoms continue even after rest you should consult your doctor.

Manage your weight

Obesity has become a major health concern worldwide, 65% of adults in US are overweight. And in case of children aged 2 to 19 one third of them are obese.

If you are overweight or obese then weight loss is the most effective lifestyle changes for controlling blood pressure. Even losing a small weight of 10 pounds (4.5 kilograms) can help reduce your blood pressure. One study with 181 overweight and hypertensive patients for 4 years showed that even if you lose only 10% of weight blood pressure is reduced 3 to 4 points.

There are many online calculators available to measure your BMI (Body Mass Index).

You can use the following site to calculate your BMI
https://www.nhlbi.nih.gov/health/educational/lose_wt/BMI/bmical c.htm

Body mass index (BMI) is an estimation of body fat based on height and weight of adults. BMI between 25 and 30 is considered overweight, over 30 is considered obese. Overweight or Obesity increases load on the heart, blood cholesterol and triglyceride levels increases, and HDL (good) cholesterol levels lowers. All of these causes your blood pressure to rise.

Being overweight can also cause disrupted breathing while you sleep, a condition called sleep apnea, which further raises your blood pressure.

Distribution of Fat in your body also has a role. Fat distribution in the abdominal trunk is called abdominal obesity. Abdominal obesity is defined by a waist circumference greater that 102 cm (40in) for men and 88 cm (35 in) for women. Abdominal obesity has the greatest influence on developing hypertension.

Calculate your body mass index and consult your doctor   to manage your weight. Use specific diet and exercise recommended by your doctor to lose weight and to control high blood pressure.

Studies show if you lose weight and achieve normal blood pressure you may not need to continue medicine to control your blood pressure. Sometimes if you reach ideal body weight with normal blood pressure your ongoing medicine will be stopped by your doctor.

Medicines used in Hypertension

The most concern about every medicine we take is side effect. As drugs of hypertension needs to be taken a long time sometimes all your life we worry about the side effects more. Is it possible to avoid drugs completely? The answer is complicated. Control of high blood pressure needs multiple factors. It is proven that lifestyle modification and modifying your diet can control high blood pressure. But to control stage 2 and stage 3 hypertension medicine is essential.

Another important aspect of hypertension medicines is prevention of complication. Most of the time medicine is given to keep the cardiovascular system (Heart, blood vessels) healthy and to stop damage. They prevent premature ageing of the cardiovascular system. In reality the main goal of hypertension medicine is to prevent, not to control blood pressure.

We have many kinds of hypertension medicine working on different mechanisms to control blood pressure. Hypertension treatment with drugs is different from other treatment. Blood pressure medicine needs individual adjustment of dose. The choice of drug is also individualized. Initially you may have to go through a trial and error phase to find the right drug and perfect dose. Don't be alarmed if your doctor frequently changes your drug or dose initially. We take several factors to choose the antihypertensive medicine. Such as

- Your general health
- Sex
- Age
- Severity of the high blood pressure;
- Any additional, underlying medical condition
- Potential side effects

If you have Bronchial asthma, heart disease, diabetes or gout. In these conditions, certain drugs are especially good, but others may be contraindicated.

The medicine on which you will respond depends on factors such as:

- The causes of your high blood pressure.
- How high your blood pressure is.
- How your body responds to different high blood pressure medicines.
- Any other health problems such as diabetes or high cholesterol you might have.

Most drugs for lowering high blood pressure are effective upto 24 hours so, most of the time one tablet taken in the morning or night is enough to control high blood pressure. But when high blood pressure is severe or resistant to treatment, more than one tablet may be needed. Some of us may need three or more drugs to control blood pressure. There is evidence that low doses of two blood pressure lowering drugs are more effective than either given alone. Moreover, low dose of two drugs causes less side effect.

There may be some trial and error testing to find the combination of high blood pressure medicine that works best for you. Many people need more than one type of high blood pressure medicine in order to get the best results. Your doctor will decide which one is best for you. Choosing the best medicine may need some trial and error, do not be alarmed if initially your doctor changes drug or dose too often.

You need to have a treatment goal if you are taking or consider taking medicines for Hypertension. The treatment goal depends on your age, health status and if you have another disease such as diabetes.

- As a general rule 120 /80 mm Hg or lower is the recommended blood pressure goal.
- If you are a healthy adult with age 60 or more your goal should be Less than150/90 mm Hg.
- Less than140/90 mm Hg is recommended If you're a healthy adult younger than age 60
- If you have chronic kidney disease, diabetes or coronary artery disease or are at high risk of coronary artery disease your goal should be Less than140/90 mm Hg.

We always worry about taking any medicine for their side effects. As we have to take hypertension medicines for a long time considering safety of the medicine is very important. But you need not to worry. Medicines treating high blood pressure is extensively tested for their safety in long time use. In reality, not taking medicines may harm you more than the mild side effects. The side effects depend upon the specific drug given, dose, and other factors.

Although antihypertensive drugs are generally well tolerated, still they have some side effects;

Some of the time when starting High blood pressure medicines for the first time, it may lower blood pressure abruptly. This sudden low blood pressure may cause dizziness, drowsiness, lightheadedness, or feeling of fainting with sudden movement. These symptoms usually subside after a few weeks.

Following are the common medicines used to treat high blood pressure along with information on their safety and side effects.

Diuretics

If you need medicine for hypertension diuretics are used as a first choice. Diuretics are a class of drugs. They work on the kidneys and wash out more salt and water from the body. Removing water results in less blood volume circulating in your blood vessels. Less volume means heart works less with less force, leading to lower blood pressure. Diuretics remove water from your body through urine so there is an increase in frequency and volume of urine. That's why they are called "water pills".

There are many drugs in the class diuretics. For hypertension, most used one is thiazide diuretics. The following drugs are classified as diuretics;

- Furosemide
- Torasemide
- Eplerenone
- Spironolactone
- Triamterene
- Amiloride
- Bendroflumethiazide
- Chlortalidone
- Cyclopenthiazide
- Indapamide
- Metolazone
- Xipamide
- Bumetanide

Sometimes you may need a combination of two diuretics to control hypertension. Some examples of combination diuretics are:

- Spironolactone and Hydrochlorothiazide
- Hydrochlorothiazide and Triamterene
- Amiloride hydrochloride and Hydrochlorothiazide

Usually for most of the people there is no side effect of hypertension medicine. A few of us may have mild side effects. The side effects usually occur when trying new drug or increased dose.

Most of the time these side effects subside over time. If you feel the side effects for a long time, then you may need to change the drug.

Possible side-effects of -diuretic include:

- An increased need to go to the toilet (Increased Urine)
- Feeling thirsty
- Feeling dizzy, weak, lethargic or sick
- Low blood pressure when moving from lying or sitting to standing
- Muscle cramps
- Skin rash
- Increase complications of Gout due to increased uric acid levels
- Increased blood glucose levels
- Erectile Dysfunction in men.

The important side effect of Diuretics is it may lower the amount of potassium in your body. Low potassium in blood is termed as hypokalemia. It is a dangerous condition. Your doctor will monitor your potassium level in blood from time to time.

Things you need to be careful when taking diuretics are;

- You should take your diuretic in the morning as they produce more urine than normal. This will help you avoid having to get up in the night to go to the toilet frequently.
- You need to have regular blood and urine tests to check potassium and blood sugar levels.
- Thiazide diuretic with beta-blocker increase risk of developing diabetes. Make sure you are not taking them together.
- Check with your doctor before taking any other medicines, including over the counter drugs.

Beta-Blockers

Beta blockers are a group of drug work by blocking the effects of the hormone epinephrine, also known as adrenaline. This hormone (epinephrine/ adrenaline) increases heart rate and constrict blood vessels. When you take beta blockers the action of the hormone is blocked, your heart beats more slowly and with less force, thereby reducing blood pressure. Beta blockers also help blood vessels to relax, which improve blood flow.

Beta blockers are not the first choice in treating hypertension. If other drugs as diuretics could not control your hypertension Beta blockers are used. Most of the time Beta blocker is used in combination of two or more drugs. Combination may include angiotensin-converting enzyme (ACE) inhibitors, diuretics or calcium channel blockers.

Beta blocked is relatively safe for long term use. Some side effects happen with Beta blocker which is mild and does not carry a risk to your health.

- Common side effects of beta blockers include:
  - Fatigue
  - Cold hands or feet
  - Weight gain
- Less common side effects include:
  - Shortness of breath
  - Trouble sleeping
  - Depression

Generally, Beta blockers are not used in people with asthma because it can trigger severe asthma attacks. In people who have diabetes, beta blockers may hide signs of low blood sugar, such as rapid heartbeat. You need to monitor your blood sugar regularly while on Beta blocker. Beta blockers can slightly increase triglyceride level in blood. And a modest decrease may occur in HDL (high-density lipoprotein) which is the good cholesterol.

Beta blockers may not work effectively for black and older people, especially when taken without other blood pressure medications.

You shouldn't abruptly stop taking a beta blocker because doing so could increase your risk of a heart attack or other heart problems. When taking beta blockers, you should

- Beta blocker lowers the heart rate. You need to learn to check your pulse. Check your pulse regularly to make sure your heart rate is not too slow (less than 60).
- Beta blockers sometimes cause higher blood sugar levels. On the other hand, beta-blockers can hide your symptoms of low blood sugar. You need to be alert if you are a diabetic taking betablockers.

Alpha-blockers for Hypertension

Blood vessels of our body have a muscle layer responsible for regulation of blood flow. There are receptor present in all the muscles. These receptors work like buttons, when they are activated muscles tighten leading to tightening of blood vessels. Then heart has to work hard with more force causing high blood pressure.

Alpha blockers block these specific receptors so receptors can't be activated leading to lower blood pressure.

Alpha-blockers are usually the third or fourth choice to control blood pressure. Because alpha blockers can only lower blood pressure, they don't have protective ability to protect and prevent heart attack or stroke, like other blood pressure medicine. Most of the time alpha blocker is used in combination of two or more drugs.

Alpha blockers used to treat high blood pressure include:

- Doxazosin
- Prazosin
- Terazosin

If you are starting Alpha Blocker for the first time you need to take the first dose at bedtime. Alpha Blocker causes a marked low blood pressure initially so you may experience dizziness and feeling of fainting or may faint when move suddenly (e.g. suddenly standing from toilet). This effect is called first dose effect and will subside after some time. So initially take Alpha Blocker before going to bed.

Other side effects of alpha blocker include:

- Headache
- Pounding heartbeat
- Weakness
- Dizziness
- Weight gain

Alpha blockers can increase or decrease the effects of other medications Such as beta blockers, calcium channel blockers or medications for erectile dysfunction. Before taking an alpha blocker, remember to inform your doctor if you are taking other medicines.

Alpha blocker is avoided in women because they can cause stress incontinence and loss of bladder control. If you are pregnant, breastfeeding or planning a pregnancy, do not take alpha blockers. Alpha Blocker is avoided in patients of heart failure, liver disease or decreased kidney function. Alpha Blocker is not given Parkinson's' disease.

Possible side-effects of alpha-blockers include:

- Sudden drops in blood pressure when -sitting up or standing up
- Headaches with nausea
- Swollen legs or ankles
- Tremor
- Rash or itchiness of the skin
- Problems with erections in men.

ACE inhibitors

Normal blood pressure is regulated in our body by some mechanism. One of these mechanisms is by a hormone called Angiotensin. Angiotensin tightens blood vessel and increase pressure. Angiotensin Converting Enzyme (ACE) inhibitors are a class of high blood pressure medicine which prevents our body from making angiotensin II from Angiotensin.

Angiotensin converting enzyme (ACE) inhibitors relax or open up the blood vessels to improve circulation blood and lower blood pressure. ACE inhibitors also decrease the amount of work your heart has to do. Examples of ACE inhibitors include:

- Captopril
- Enalapril
- Lisinopril
- Benazepril
- Fosinopril
- Ramipril
- Quinapril
- Perindopril
- Trandolapril
- Moexipril

ACE inhibitor drugs are given as a first choice if you need medicine to control your blood pressure. They are the drug of choice for young people (less than 55 years of age) who developed hypertension.

Like any drug, an ACE inhibitors have some side effects. They may include:

- Cough. Some people not in everyone ACE inhibitors cause a persistent dry cough. If you get it than you have to stop this class of drugs.
- ACE inhibitors may cause red, itchy skin or rash.
- Sudden change of posture like standing from sitting position you may feel dizziness, lightheadedness or fainting. It is due to sudden fall of blood pressure.
- A salty & metallic taste or a reduced ability to taste.
- You may experience some physical symptoms such as sore throat, mouth sores, fast or irregular heartbeat, chest pain, and swelling of feet, ankles and lower legs. It can also cause Swelling of your neck, face, and tongue. You need to consult your doctor immediately if you experience these symptoms. These symptoms may represent a serious emergency.
- ACE inhibitors can cause high potassium levels in the blood called as hyperkalemia. This is a potentially life-threatening complication. You should regularly check your potassium level in blood.

  High potassium in blood or Hyperkalemia is a dangerous condition, there are some symptoms associated with high potassium such as irregular heartbeat, tingling and numbness in hand, foot or around lips. It may cause confusion, drowsiness and breathing problem. Be alert for these symptoms. Seek immediate potassium level check and treatment if the symptoms show up.

Some Guidelines for Taking ACE Inhibitors

- Always take ACE inhibitors on an empty stomach one hour before meals.
- Monitor your blood pressure and kidney function regularly when on ACE Inhibitor.
- Salt substitute contains high potassium so do not use salt substitutes while taking ACE Inhibitors. You need to read food labels to choose low-sodium and low-potassium foods.
- You cannot take ACE inhibitors during pregnancy. They can cause death or deformity in the newborn
- ACE inhibitor can pass through breast milk so avoid it if you breast feed your baby.

Calcium Channel Blockers

Another class of drug used to control blood pressure is called Calcium Channel Blockers (CCB). For the pumping action heart muscles need calcium ions. CCB blocks the pathway of calcium ions. So, heart muscle gets calcium slowly. Heart stays relaxed. CCB also widens blood vessels so heart has to work less all these helps to lower blood pressure to normal level.

Examples of calcium channel blockers include:

- Amlodipine
- Felodipine
- Isradipine
- Nicardipine
- Nifedipine
- Diltiazem
- Nimodipine
- Verapamil

Possible side-effects of calcium-channel blockers include:

- Swollen ankles
- Ankle or foot pain
- Constipation
- Skin rashes
- A flushed face
- Headaches
- Dizziness or tiredness
- Swollen or bleeding gums (rarely)

If you are taking a calcium-channel blocker you should not drink grapefruit juice. Grapefruit juice makes absorption of CCB rapidly and more. With more drug in your blood cause blood pressure to drop suddenly and dangerously low level.

Calcium Channel Blockers are not used If there is kidney or liver disease along with hypertension.

Angiotensin II Receptor Blockers (ARB)

As I have mentioned earlier a hormone called Angiotensin helps regulate blood pressure. Angiotensin binds with receptors present in blood vessels and tighten them. Angiotensin Receptor Blockers (ARB) block these receptors keeping the blood vessels relaxed with smooth blood flow, in effect blood pressure lowers to a normal level.

Angiotensin II receptor blockers include:

- Valsartan
- Candesartan
- Eprosartan
- Irbesartan
- Losartan

- Olmesartan
- Telmisartan
- Valsartan

ARB is the first choice if you need two or more combined blood pressure medicine. For younger patients (age less than 55 years), diabetic patients and patients of kidney disease ARB is the drug of choice. ARB has a protective role on kidneys.

If you are pregnant, breastfeeding or planning a pregnancy, you should not be given an angiotensin receptor blocker. Because angiotensin II receptor blockers can injure a developing fetus.

Very few people have side effects with ARB. Possible side effects include:

- Dizziness
- Increased potassium level in blood (hyperkalemia)
- Swelling of tissues (angioedema)
- Diarrhea
- Gross weight loss

Direct Vasodilators

This class of high blood pressure medicine works on blood vessels directly. They relax the muscles in your blood vessel walls. This makes the blood vessels to widen and blood flows through them more easily. This results in lower blood pressure.

Direct vasodilators are:

- Hydralazine
- Minoxidil

Usually these drugs are used in resistant hypertension when three or more drugs are needed to control blood pressure. They are also used in hypertensive emergency.

Usually direct vasodilator is used in combination with a diuretic and a beta blocker.

Direct vasodilators have some side effect such as rapid heartbeat, headaches and joint pain.

Central Agonists

Our body has amazing mechanisms to maintain our blood pressure in normal level. One of the mechanism maintains blood pressure by increasing or decreasing heart rate using signals from our brain. Centrally acting drugs binds with the receptor present in our brain and activate them. Active receptors send signal to the heart to slow down. Lower heart rate decreases the blood pressure. It also causes to relax our blood vessels.

Central Agonists include:

- Methyldopa
- Clonidine
- Guanfacine
- Guanabenz

Due to strong side effects these drugs are usually not used. Side effects include:

- Fatigue
- Drowsiness or sedation
- Dizziness
- Impotence
- Constipation
- Abnormally slow heart rate
- Dry mouth
- Headache
- Fever

If you are taking Central Agonist never stop the drug suddenly. When central agonists are stopped abruptly it causes a sudden and very high rise in blood pressure, which is very dangerous.

Direct Renin Inhibitors

Direct Renin Inhibitors are new drugs for hypertension. How does it work! You may be surprised to know that normal blood pressure level is maintained by our kidneys. Kidneys produce an enzyme called "Renin" which has an active role in regulating blood pressure. Direct renin inhibitors block renin to work. Without the trigger event of renin our blood vessels stay relaxed and wide. Blood flows smoothly causing blood pressure to decrease.

Tekturna is a direct renin inhibitor. As high blood pressure medicine, Tekturna is used alone or in combination other medicines.

As direct renin inhibitors are a new type of medicine for high blood pressure. Studies are ongoing to know about the safety of the drug after prolonged use.

Take direct renin inhibitors only if prescribed by your doctor.

Peripheral-Acting Adrenergic Blockers

Peripheral adrenergic blockers as the name implies blocks nerve impulse. By this blocking muscles in our blood vessels relaxes. Less force then needed by heart to keep blood flowing. In turn the blood pressure decreases.

Peripheral acting adrenergic blockers include:

- Guanadrel

- Guanethidine
- Reserpine

These medicines are usually not used. If other medicines including combined medicines fail to control blood pressure, then these drugs are used.

Medicine for Specific Conditions

Some specific conditions need specific blood pressure medicine. These recommended medicines have been proved by large studies showing more benefit than other drugs. For example;

- Diabetic patients with hypertension response more with Angiotensin Converting Enzyme (ACE) Inhibitor. Beside controlling blood pressure ACE inhibitors protects kidney and heart specially in diabetic patients.
- The drug class Beta blockers work best for people with heart failure and heart attack. They prevent heart attack beside controlling blood pressure.
- Along with lowering high blood pressure Calcium Channel Blockers control symptoms in people with angina caused by poor blood supply to heart muscles due to coronary artery disease.

Also, there are some antihypertensive drugs that should not be used in certain conditions. Such as;

- ACE inhibitors and angiotensin II receptor blockers (ARBs) must be avoided during pregnancy and breast feeding.
- Gout patients should not get the drugs classified as diuretics or water pills. They can worsen gout.

Combination of medicine

Combination drug therapy — Sometimes and in some people lifestyle modification along with a single medicine could not control blood pressure. Then a combination of two or more drugs used together. Treating high blood pressure needs individualized drug and dose adjustment. So if you're given a combination of drugs don't be worried it's a recommended treatment protocol.

Sometimes If a person has very high blood pressure (eg, 160/100 mmHg or higher), then combination therapy with two or more drugs can be started from the very beginning of treatment.

The beneficial side of combination therapy are

- They may be more effective than increasing the dose of the single drug
- Amazingly a combination of drugs has less side effect than a single drug with higher doses.

Acupuncture for Hypertension

Usually Acupuncture is not used as a treatment of Hypertension. In specific situations, you may try acupuncture with supervision of your doctor or licensed acupuncture professional.

Acupuncture is a 3000 years old treatment practice originating from China. It is used for treating many diseases. In Europe, Canada and western world treatment using acupuncture started 100 years ago, but it becomes popular and widespread rapidly in the second half of twentieth century. In 1996 US regulators approved acupuncture as a treatment by licensed professionals. According to World Health Organization(WHO) acupuncture is effective for treatment of 28 conditions. Mild to moderate Hypertension can be treated with acupuncture.

Traditional Chinese medicine and acupuncture explains that "Health is the harmonious balance of YIN and YANG. It is believed imbalance between Yin and Yang causes diseases. According Chinese medicine our life force is CHI, and it floats through our body via specific points called meridians. Through 350 meridian points of the body we can access this life force. If acupuncture needle is inserted at specific meridian points it can restore the balance of Yin and Yang. By restoring balance acupuncture cure diseases.

The medical community throughout the world does not agree on how acupuncture works. By western practitioner the meridian points are seen as nerve ending, muscle or connective tissue. By acupuncture needle these nerves or tissue can be stimulated. Which in turn increase blood flow to the area. Acupuncture creates nerve impulse causing pain killer effect or other effect to cure the disease.

On the effect of acupuncture on hypertension very few studies are done. There is a small study conducted at the University of California Irvine(UCI) on the effect of acupuncture on hypertension.

The study shows 70% of the study group shows a noticeable drop in blood pressure. On average systolic blood pressure dropped 6 to 8 mm/Hg, and 4 mm/Hg drop occurred in diastolic blood pressure. And these improvements were persistent for 6 weeks after the treatment. Noradrenalin a hormone and Renin an enzyme of our body causes high blood pressure. Acupuncture also shows 4% drop in noradrenalin and a 67% drop in renin.

According to study reduction of high blood pressure were clinically significant and useful for patients 60 or more years of age with systolic hypertension (age related hypertension).

Risk factors of Acupuncture

- The risk of complication from acupuncture is low. But you must seek a certified acupuncture practitioner. Some complication such as Soreness, Minor bleeding, can occur.
- There is a chance of injury to internal organs such as lungs, heart or spinal cord but it's extremely rare.
- You can get infected if the needles are not properly sterilized. There is a chance of transmission of disease such as Hepatitis B or C, HIV etc.

In some condition acupuncture, should not be done

- If you have any type of bleeding disorder you should not try acupuncture. There is some medicine used in thinning of blood such as Warfarin causes prolonged bleeding so acupuncture is contraindicated.
- If you have a pacemaker, then do not try acupuncture specially acupuncture with electric impulse.
- If you are pregnant acupuncture is contraindicated.

Natural or Herbal remedies for Hypertension

You will find literally thousand home remedies for Hypertension. There are many medicinal plants used as herbal or natural medicine controlling high blood pressure throughout the world. The problem with home remedies or herbal treatment is that most of the home remedies or herbal treatment has no study or data or has very small study to backup their claims. Study and research are still ongoing to evaluate most of the herbal remedies.

There is a common belief or myth that herbal medicine or Home remedies do not have any side effects or they are safer than other treatment. It's not completely true. To find out the side effect or adverse effect of any medicine we need large studies over a long period but most of the herbal remedies has no proper study. Following herbal remedies need more study before labeling them as safe from side effects;

- Rauwolfia serpentina (snakeroot)
- Stephania tetrandra (tetrandrine)
- Panax notoginseng (ginseng)
- Crataegus species (hawthorn)

Some herbal treatment has proven toxic effect on liver (Hepatotoxic) and Kidneys(Nephrotoxic) in large doses.

Some study show that following herbal remedies may increase blood pressure, so if you have hypertension you need to avoid them.

- Licorice
- Yohimbine
- Ephedra (Ma Huang)

Because of potential health risks associated with these herbs, it is important that you inform your doctor if you plan to use or are already using herbal treatment. When some of these herbs are used in combination with high blood pressure drugs it may potentiate or reduce the effects of medicine. They may increase the side effects of drugs when used together. Following are some commonly used home or natural remedies claimed to lower your blood pressure.

Hibiscus Tea for High Blood Pressure

Hibiscus is a beautiful tropical plant. Its scientific name is Hibiscus sabdariffa. Hibiscus tea is prepared by using parts of the hibiscus plant mainly the flower. Hibiscus flowers have various local names, "Roselle" is another commonly used name of hibiscus. Most of the commercial herbal tea blends in the United States contain hibiscus.

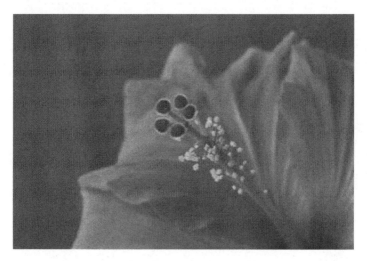

Hibiscus tea is used to lower high blood pressure throughout the world. It is a popular medicinal drink preferred by natural medicine practitioners. It contains anthocyanins in high concentration. Anthocyanins inhibit angiotensin-converting enzyme (ACE) and in turn lower blood pressure. The claim is yet to be proved by large study.

There are some small studies done on hibiscus tea. These studies show hibiscus tea lower high blood pressure. One of the study is done by Diane L. McKay, PhD, of Tufts University in Boston. The study shows, "drinking three cups of herbal tea containing hibiscus each day lowered systolic blood pressure by an average of 7 points. That was significantly more than the 1 point drop observed in people who were given hibiscus-flavored water as placebo".

In general Hibiscus is safe. You can take it as a drink in adequate amount. But it is Unsafe during pregnancy. There is evidence that hibiscus might cause a miscarriage. Based on the research held at the Guru Jambheshwar University of Science and Technology in India. One study concluded that "excessive consumption of hibiscus tea reduces women fertility and effects childbearing. Hibiscus tea might reduce the level of estrogen and effect women's reproductive ability". So, if you are women avoid hibiscus or herbal tea containing hibiscus completely there is other safe alternative available. There is not enough reliable information or study on the safety of taking hibiscus while breastfeeding. To stay on the safe side, and avoid it during breastfeeding.

Hibiscus might decrease blood sugar levels. Keep monitoring your blood glucose when taking hibiscus tea. If there is frequent low blood sugar, then you need to adjust the dose of your diabetes medications. It is best to consult your doctor.

Apple cider Vinegar for Hypertension

One of the common food people use and suggest to lower high blood pressure is "Apple cider Vinegar". You must have heard or read on internet about Apple cider vinegar and its effectiveness on high blood pressure. Some claim apple cider vinegar is the best natural medicine for health, hypertension and circulatory control.

The problem is there is no significant study done on Apple Cider Vinegar and its effect on hypertension. Some studies are done on the effect of ACV on diabetes which shows ACV can help with diabetes and weight loss (Study in Japan with 175 people). Another interesting thing with ACV is its nutritional value is very low. Normally It does not contain any vitamins (like vitamin A, B, C or E). It does not contain nutritional elements like amino acid, lycopene etc.

We still do not know how ACV may work. There are some hypothesis. According to one hypothesis Apple pectin is a natural circulatory health boost. Apple pectin may help body to clean veins and arteries. Vinegar is very acidic, so when taken your body speeds up the metabolic process to get the vinegar out of the stomach. This process may boost your metabolism. With high metabolic rate your body needs more energy leading to weight loss and control obesity. This also helps in weight loss, because as your speeds up to boost itself, using carbohydrate. But keep in mind there is no major research done to find out how ACV may work. There is very limited study or proof that AVC work as a wonder cure all natural medicine.

Hypertension medicines need individual adjustment that means you may respond to a treatment different than others. So, you can try Apple cider vinegar with monitoring of blood pressure. If you plan to give Apple Cider Vinegar(ACV) a try go ahead, but do not stop your prescribed medicines. It's better if you consult with your doctor first.

Don't take ACV straight, its acidic and may harm your esophagus and   tooth   enamel. Don't take a lot of ACV. Take 2 tablespoon with water 2 to 3 times a day with food. There is pills/capsule containing ACV is available over the counter. You may take those if you don't like the taste of ACV.

Garlic for Hypertension

Garlic is scientifically known as *Allium sativum*, is a species of the onion genus. Garlic is extensively used as natural medicine thousands of years. It is used to treat various diseases or condition in India, China and Egypt, also in Germany and in countries all over the world where garlic is not readily available.

Medicinal use of garlic has various applications. But it's mostly used in cardiovascular conditions and to control high levels of fat (Lipids) in your blood called hyperlipidemia. Research shows that when garlic is taken by mouth for a few months it can reduce blood pressure by as much as 7% or 8% in people with moderately high blood pressure. A 2013 meta-analysis concluded that "garlic preparations may effectively lower total cholesterol by 11–23 mg/dL and LDL cholesterol by 3–15 mg/dL in adults with high cholesterol if taken for longer than two months". By reducing cholesterol garlic helps to complications of high blood pressure.

Garlic contains a biologically active substance called allicin and garlic sulphides. Garlic works by three mechanisms. Allicin of garlic relaxes blood vessels, maintains a smooth flow reducing blood pressure and vessel damage. It also blocks the function of angiotensin to keep blood vessels relaxed and wide. Garlic also activates the production of nitric oxide synthesis which helps relax blood vessels.

If you want to control blood pressure with natural products, if you want to avoid hypertension drugs then you should try Garlic first. Most likely it will lower blood pressure to a normal level.

Garlic is safe for most people when taken by mouth appropriately an in small amount. It can be taken for a long time. Garlic has been used safely in research for up to 7 years without any side effect.

There are some minor side effects in some people. When taken by mouth, garlic can cause

- Burning sensation in the mouth or stomach.
- Heartburn.

- Abdominal bloating.
- Sometimes nausea, vomiting, and diarrhea.

These side effects are often worse with raw garlic. If you experience any of these, you may switch to Garlic Capsule available over the counter.

Garlic is known to cause bad breath (halitosis) and body odor, a pungent "garlicky" smell to sweat. This is caused by allyl methyl sulfide (AMS) present in garlic. AMS is a volatile liquid which is absorbed into the blood from stomach. Then via blood it travels to the lungs. As it is a volatile substance it is expelled by respiration causing bad breath. Some garlic products are made "odorless" by aging the garlic, but this makes garlic less effective. You may take supplements that are coated so they dissolve in the intestine instead of stomach. If you want to try garlic be sure to consult your partner first. Your partner will be suffered with your bad breath and garlicky body odor!

For individual dose consult your doctor.

Food supplements for hypertension

There are certain food supplements claiming to reduce hypertension. Most of the supplements do not have sufficient studies to confirm their claims. Some studies show promising results.

Coenzyme Q10 (CoQ10)

Coenzyme Q10 is a naturally occurring enzyme of our body. Studies at the University of Texas and in Osaka, Japan, showed a very promising result. It showed that if 45 to 60 mg of CoQ10 taken daily it lowered blood pressure levels 12 to 25 points or more. In the study, patients of moderate high blood pressure CoQ10 alone without any medicine reduced blood pressure in normal level.

Coenzyme Q10 has other beneficial effects. It helps maintain circulatory health by keeping heart muscle and blood vessels healthy.

Omega-3 fatty acids

There are some essential fatty acids that our body needs. As our body, can't make them we have to get it from our diet. Omega-3 fatty acid is one of these essential fatty acids.

Several clinical studies suggest that Omega3 has a positive effect on heart and blood vessels. It also lower blood pressure in hypertensive patients. An analysis of 17 clinical studies using fish oil supplements as a source of Omega3, found that taking 3 or more grams of fish daily reduce blood pressure in people with hypertension.

Modest reductions of blood pressure may occur with significantly higher doses 3 or more grams of omega-3 fatty acids. But more than 3 gm of Omega 3 increase the risk of bleeding. So don't take more than 3 gm.

The American Heart Association (AHA) recommends that "you should eat fish (particularly fatty, cold water fish) at least twice a week". Other fish containing a rich source of Omega 3are Salmon, mackerel, herring, sardines, lake trout, and tuna. The AHA says taking up to 3 or less than 3 grams of fish oil daily in supplement form is safe.

Side effects from omega-3 fish oil may include:

- A fishy taste in your mouth
- Fishy breath
- Abdominal distension and discomfort
- Loose stools
- Nausea

Amino Acids for Hypertension

Amino acids are essential for our body to function. Amino acids are made by our body. But we can also get them through food. Some studies suggest specific amino acid L-arginine & L-taurine may lower blood pressure. Then again, some studies show that L arginine works for a very short period. Blood pressure may become high after some time. There is no large enough study done to confirm the effect of L-arginine. The effect of L-taurine on high blood pressure is also yet to be proven by large study.

Our body makes sufficient quantity of L-arginine for our need. Usually we don't need to take them as a supplement. In some condition, such as diabetes may cause deficiency then we need to take L-arginine. It is available in nuts, fish, red meat, soy, whole grains, beans and dairy products. It's also available as supplements. It is believed that L-arginine works on blood vessels to keep them relaxed and allow smoother flow.

Homeopathy for Hypertension

Homeopathy, also known as homeopathic medicine, is an alternative medical system that was developed in Germany more than 200 years ago, It is based on a series of ideas developed in the 1790s by a German doctor called Samuel Hahnemann.

Homeopathy is based on two unconventional theories:

- "Like cures like" means that a disease can be cured by a substance that produces similar symptoms in healthy people.
- "Law of minimum dose" means that the lower the dose of the medication, the greater its effectiveness.

There is little evidence to support homeopathy as an effective treatment for any specific condition. Homeopathy does not relate with fundamental laws of chemistry. Some homeopathic medicine does not contain any active ingredient so there is no possibility of any effect. The effect of homeopathy can be explained scientifically by an effect called "Placebo effect". In placebo effect a patient may experience cure or improvement of symptoms without any medicine if he believes and take some pills or treatment given by doctors.

Problem with research or study homeopathic treatment is difficult because homeopathic treatments are highly individualized, and there is no uniform prescribing standard or common guideline for homeopathic practitioners. There are hundreds of different homeopathic remedies, which can be prescribed in a variety of different dilutions for thousands of symptoms.

All this information indicates that you should not take homeopathic treatment for hypertension. But if you still want to give it a try, consult with your doctor first.

Meditation for Hypertension

Anxiety, stress or tension can cause a sudden increase in blood pressure. During stress a hormone called Adrenaline increase in our body. Adrenaline increases the heart rate leading to increased blood pressure. They are also responsible for other dangerous conditions such as stroke and heart attack.

Meditation is a thousand years old practice. We have used meditation since the dawn of medical science developed by shamans. And studies have proven that this ancient treatment works on many conditions. In modern times, new methods of meditation are being developed for specific conditions. For high blood pressure a specific type of meditation called "Transendal Meditation" works best.

Usually in meditation we use deep breath with focusing on tranquility of mind. It causes a deep relaxation without sleep and removes stress from our mind. In Transendal meditation uses deep breathing with a focus on any color or sound or peaceful memory to concentrate.

Recent studies have offered promising results about the impact of Transendal Meditation in reducing blood pressure. A 2012 study (in African American 5 year follow up) showed that with Transendal Meditation the risk of heart attack or stroke is 48% reduced.

In Transendal medicine you need a quiet environment. Some soothing music or sound can be used. You can also focus on your heart beat or respiration. You need to be seated with your eyes closed. Then focus on any music, sound or a peaceful memory. Relax yourself don't work too hard on focusing. You need to do this for 15 to 20 minutes, best if done twice a day.

Studies have shown meditation is very effective in reducing easing stress. We think the deep relaxed state of meditation may start biochemical changes beneficial to the body. It may trigger the self-healing capacity of our body. It restores the balance between our mind and body.

There are countless types of meditation, so start anything that you are comfortable with. Try some different types of meditation to what works for you.

Prayer is also a powerful form of mediation.

PART THREE
ANSWER TO QUESTIONS THAT YOU MAY ASK

Following are answers to some common questions all of us want to know. Some questions we always want to ask but too silly or embarrassing for us to really ask it are included. I request my readers to send me more questions to be included in future editions of this book. If you have any question on hypertension no matter how silly it may sound send it to dr.shahriar@doctor.com

What is hypertension

Blood pressure is the force of blood against our blood vessels as it circulates. This force is necessary to make the blood flow, delivering nutrients and oxygen throughout the body. Our heart pumps and creates this flow.

Medically High blood pressure is called hypertension, means there is more pressure on our blood vessels.

Which blood pressure Is more dangerous: systolic or diastolic?

The common belief that diastolic pressure is more significant than systolic is not true. Both systolic and diastolic high blood pressure significantly increases the risk of cardiovascular disease. Newer studies show "Especially in people above 50, systolic hypertension is   more   dangerous   than   diastolic".

Is isolated systolic pressure dangerous?

For years, doctors focused primarily on diastolic blood pressure. Previously we thought high systolic pressure is manageable by the body and high diastolic pressure is responsible for complications of hypertension. Studies have proven it wrong. Studies have shown that systolic pressure is as important as diastolic pressure. And in elderly people (age more than 50) systolic pressure is more important.

For people age 50 or more systolic pressure may rise without any change in diastolic pressure. This is called isolated systolic hypertension. It needs treatment.

Without any specific condition, such as diabetes, obesity, hardening of the arteries (atherosclerosis), or a history of heart disease or a heart attack some increase in diastolic pressure (more than 95) does not have any significant health risk.

Is hypertension inevitable?

No. Hypertension is not inevitable. It is a common misconception that "Every one of us will get hypertension, maybe in the later part of our life". Recent data and studies show high blood pressure does not occur in all of us, even if we reach the risky age of 65 and more.

So, hypertension is not inevitable.

You may be at an increased risk for getting high blood pressure if you smoke, are overweight, eat a diet that's low on fiber and high in fat and salt, drink alcohol to excess, live with chronic stress or don't get much physical activity. Your lifetime risk of developing high blood pressure may be a dangerous 90% or more but still it's not 100% or inevitable.

Is Hypertension natural result of aging?

Rise in the blood pressure is a natural result of ageing. With the aging process, blood vessels naturally stiffen. As the blood vessels stiffens its flexibility is lost. The amount of force required to pump blood through arteries increases and it results in more pressure against artery walls.

Due to ageing blood pressure rise in a specific way. Particularly systolic blood pressure naturally rises with age. The diastolic blood pressure stays at a same level upto 50 years of age. Then diastolic pressure usually begins to decline slowly over 50 years of age. After 50 years of age diastolic pressure slowly declines. This specific type of hypertension occurring after 50 years of age is called isolated systolic hypertension. More than 90% of adults develops Isolated systolic hypertension in their lifetime.

Fortunately, high blood pressure in most cases, easy to control. And that's why it's so critical to monitor your blood pressure regularly.

How to read blood pressure measurement?

There are two components in blood pressure reading. Such as 117 slash 76 mm Hg, read as "117 over 76 millimeters of mercury"

The higher number is systolic blood pressure it indicates the highest level of force against the artery wall. The lower number is diastolic blood pressure, it indicates the blood pressure during relaxed state of heart.

Importance of monitoring blood pressure?

Monitoring Blood pressure is important because the higher your blood pressure is, the higher is your risk of complications in future.

Long standing high blood pressure causes extra strain on your arteries and heart. Over time if uncontrolled this strain makes blood vessels thick, weaker and less flexible. These gradually causes your blood vessels to become narrow, even blocked sometimes. This results in many dangerous complications such as heart attack, stroke, kidney disease, dementia etc. Sometimes the weak vessel may burst open inside the body causing a serious life threatening health crisis.

When should I start monitoring blood pressure?

High blood pressure usually do not give symptoms so it can't be detected without being measured. If your blood pressure is below 120/80 mm Hg, still get it checked at least once every two years, starting at age 20. If your blood pressure is higher, you may need to check it more often.

High blood pressure greatly increases your risk of heart disease and stroke. If you have a family history of high blood pressure or have other risk factors such as obesity, high cholesterol, diabetes then you need to check your blood pressure regularly at least on every 6 months.

Regular blood pressure monitoring is one of the most important screenings.

What happens during 24-hour blood pressure monitoring?

A 24-hour blood pressure measurement is just the same as a normal blood pressure check. For 24 hours at a regular interval, usually every 15-30 minutes during the daytime and 30-60 minutes at night, a digital machine takes your blood pressure automatically.

 The machine is small and worn on a belt. The cuff is wrapped around your upper arm. Normally the machine is fitted at your local hospital out patients' department, although some GP may have them.

For 24 hours, you will need to keep the monitor active, even through the night. During this 24 hour period, you have to do all your regular activities as any normal day. You can't have a bath or shower or swim during this 24 hour.

 At the end of the 24 hours the device is removed All the stored data is analyzed and a diagnosis is made.

Normal ambulatory blood pressure monitoring values?

Normal 24 hours' ambulatory blood pressure value is

- During the day, less than systolic 135 and diastolic less than 85 mm of Hg
- At Night, systolic is less than 120 and diastolic is less than 70 mm of Hg
- Levels above 140/90 mm of Hg during the day and 125/75 mm Hg at night is considered as abnormal.

Downside of ambulatory blood pressure monitoring

There are some disadvantages of 24 hour blood pressure monitoring. Such as;

- It is not available everywhere, although this is improving.
- It requires specialist training.
- Some patients don't like the cuff for 24 hours.
- Sleep disturbance may occur due to inflation of the cuff every 30 minutes.
- Mild Bruising may occur where the cuff is wrapped.

- Poor technique and Arrhythmias (abnormal heart beats) may cause poor readings.

What is white coat Hypertension

Blood pressure values is not a fixed value. It rises and falls due to many causes throughout the day. It is affected by work, stress, emotional or physical work. A specific type of high blood pressure occurs in some people called white coat hypertension. In this condition when pressure is measured in a doctor's office, clinic or hospital setting blood pressure is very high. But it becomes normal when measured at home. The term "white coat" comes from references to the white coats traditionally worn by doctors.

We believe people with white coat hypertension become extremely stressed in a hospital setting, causing a sudden high blood pressure. Usually for everyone blood pressure become upto 10 points higher when measured in a hospital setting but for white coat hypertension it becomes 50 or more points higher.

What causes the white coat effect?

The usual explanation of White coat effect is that you may be very anxious and nervous about having your blood pressure measured by a doctor or nurse. We do not always notice but most of us tend to feel stressed in medical settings than we do in surroundings that are familiar to us.

The white coat effect influences some people's blood pressure more than others. If you have white coat effect your systolic blood pressure can temporarily rise by as much as 30 points or more. This makes difficult for your doctor to get an accurate measurement of your blood pressure.

How will I know I have white coat hypertension?

Anyone can be affected by the white coat effect, but white coat hypertension is not common.   The only way to be sure about the white coat effect is to compare readings taken in the clinic or doctor's office with readings taken at home. There are two ways to rule out white coat effect.

- Measure your blood pressure at home – It is best way to diagnose if you have white coat hypertension. Measure your blood pressure regularly and keep a note of your blood pressure. Your doctor may then measure blood pressure and compare home and office blood pressure levels.
- 24-hour blood pressure monitoring – Sometimes a 24 hours automatic blood pressure monitoring may be used. It shows more detailed data on your blood pressure changes throughout the day.

What can I do about white coat hypertension?

Try managing your stress before blood pressure is measured. Wait 10 to 15 minutes in a calm and quiet state before measuring. Meditation for 10 min may help greatly.

Sometimes it may not be possible to overcome the white coat effect. In this case, you need to monitor at home and keep a record of the measurement along with time. A subsequent visit of 2 to 3 times to the same doctor might help.

I have been diagnosed with high blood pressure, but could it be white coat hypertension?

If you have high blood pressure when measured at a clinic or hospital setting it may be due to white coat hypertension. To rule out your doctor will advise you 3 or more visits with blood pressure monitoring before reaching a diagnosis of hypertension.

People with white coat hypertension usually develop high blood pressure. It is important to have your blood pressure checked regularly (every 6-12 months with a medical professional).

Is white coat hypertension dangerous?

Usually in case of white coat hypertension blood pressure becomes normal. The sudden rise during measurement is not dangerous in itself. But most of the time patients with white coat hypertension develop mild to moderate hypertension later in their life. White coat hypertension is seen as an early sign of clinical hypertension by most of the physicians.

There is a possibility that due to white coat hypertension some patients get unnecessary prescribed medication to lower blood pressure. But blood pressure is in fact normal. This can cause very low blood pressure leading to generalized weakness and even unconsciousness.

To overcome this the diagnosis of hypertension is never based on a single visit. Usually there is 2 to 3 visits with multiple measurement including home measurement is used to diagnose hypertension. A 24 hours monitoring can also be used to rule out white coat hypertension.

What is home blood pressure monitoring?

When Blood Pressure (BP) is measured at doctor office or hospital there is a significant high result. So, monitoring blood pressure at home is a good choice and recommended by doctors.

For home monitoring, you need to learn how to measure blood pressure using an analog or automatic device. It's easy to learn and now available devices are almost fully automatic and very easy to operate.

What Are the Complications Associated with Essential Hypertension?

Hypertension should never be ignored. Lest untreated hypertension leads to multiple life threatening complication. As blood pressure become higher the chance of complication and severity of complication increases. Following are examples of complications of untreated hypertension;

Heart attack or Heart failure – Heart is the major organ that suffers from hypertension most. Long standing uncontrolled hypertension causes heart muscle to become thick, in time enlargement of heart occur. Enlarged heart with abnormally thickened muscle is prone to heart attack. It's a life-threatening complication of uncontrolled high blood pressure.

Atherosclerosis – Higher force of high blood pressure damage the blood vessels. Body itself repairs these vessels by depositing cells and fibers but this causes the vessels to become narrow. There is a plaque buildup inside the vessels, sometimes causing complete block of the vessels.

There is also a possibility of tearing or rupture of blood vessels. This is caused by prolonged hypertension that weakens blood vessels. Rupture of blood vessel is a medical emergency.

Kidney Disease: Hypertension can damage the small blood vessels and filters in the kidneys, so that the kidneys cannot excrete waste properly. In time, it may cause complete kidney failure.

Stroke: Uncontrolled and severe hypertension can lead to stroke, either by blocking blood vessels supplying the brain or by rupture of blood vessels caused by increased force.

Eye Disease: Hypertension can damage the very small blood vessels in eyes specifically vessels of retina which may lead to blindness.

What Is the Long-Term Outlook of hypertension?

Its true hypertension can lead to multiple complication but they only occur when hypertension is uncontrolled for a long period of time. So you need to control hypertension. There is a fair chance that you will not need any drugs, lifestyle modification along with modification of diet will keep your blood pressure checked.

If you need drugs don't be worried. Most drugs used for hypertension are studied for adverse effect or side effects for long term use. Most people don't show any side effect of hypertension medicine. Some shows mild side effects.

You need to continue your medicine lifelong even if there is no symptoms or your blood pressure is normal. Sometimes your doctor may decide to stop your medicine or lower its dose.

To prevent life threatening complication such as stroke, heart attack, kidney failure etc. You must control high blood pressure.

.

Is hypertension a Result of Aging?

A common misconception is "Hypertension occurs with age". This is not true. Blood pressure may rise with age but it may not rise to the level to diagnose as hypertension. This is proven by multiple studies. Some population in Mexico, South pacific and other part of the world show very small rise of blood pressure with age.

Is There Treatment for Prehypertension?

Prehypertension is basically a warning sign that there is a possibility of developing hypertension soon. The goal of Prehypertension is to help in wider application of lifestyle changes for the prevention of hypertension and tight monitoring of blood pressure to allow prompt treatment, if the patient develops initial stage of hypertension.

Treatment with drugs or medicines is not necessary in prehypertension stage. Lifestyle modification and modification of diet is enough to keep your blood pressure at normal levels.

Following are some strategies to help you manage prehypertension:

- Lose weight if you are overweight. Obesity leads to hypertension. You need to calculate your BMI and lose weight if necessary. By keeping ideal weight according to your height and age you can prevent high blood pressure.
- Exercise regularly. Exercise helps you lose weight. Exercise also makes your heart and blood vessels stronger to prevent prehypertension.
- Modify your diet. Eat plenty of fruits, vegetables, whole grains, fish, and low-fat dairy. Specific diet such as DASH or Pritikin can prevent and control high blood pressure.
- Limit dietary salt(sodium). Many studies have proven that a diet high in sodium (salt) can increase blood pressure. A low-sodium diet can lower high blood pressure, also prevent it. Limit salt to less than 2,300 milligrams daily (about 1 teaspoon of table salt).
- Limit Alcohol. Drink only in moderation.

It's important that you check your blood pressure regularly.

How excess salt may cause hypertension?

Salt used in our daily cooking and salt we take with food is made up of sodium chloride (NaCl). Salt in adequate amount is necessary to maintain functions of our body. Salt or sodium Chloride maintains balance of water in our body. Our kidneys wash out excess salt through urine. But daily salt (NaCl) consumption in developed countries has increased to 10 to 12 g per day. Our kidneys could not keep up the balance with this huge amount of salt. So salt along with water stays in blood increasing blood volume. This increased blood volume results in high blood pressure.

Are there any medicines that cause high blood pressure?

Some medicines available over the counter can make blood pressure rise. Also, some medications may interact with blood pressure medicine and prevent drug from working properly.

If you have hypertension you should be aware before taking any medicine. Drugs that you should be careful with hypertension include:

- Acetaminophen - Used in fever and mild pain, available as over the counter without prescription. This may increase blood pressure.
- Many over the counter cough/cold and asthma medications – may contain ephedrine or pseudoephedrine which increase your heart rate along with blood pressure.
- Nonsteroidal anti-inflammatory drugs (NSAIDs) such as Ibuprofen (Advil, Motrin), Naproxen (Aleve, Naprosyn) often

used to relieve pain may retain water causing increases in blood volume leading to increased blood pressure. These drugs can also raise your risk for heart attack or stroke, especially in higher doses.

- Caffeine including the caffeine in coffee and energy drinks increase heart rate and blood pressure.
- Estrogens available in birth control pills have an effect on blood pressure.
- Migraine medications. Some migraine medications work by tightening blood vessels. This can make blood pressure rise, even to dangerous levels.
- Nasal decongestants. Decongestants may make your blood pressure and heart rate rise due to Pseudoephedrine present in them.

So, before taking any drugs even the over the counter medicine its best to consult your doctor first.

How serious a risk is smoking for Hypertension?

The short answer is - very serious! By giving up smoking you may reduce the risk of high blood pressure to a low level. If you cannot stop smoking completely, try to reduce down to less than 10 cigarettes a day.

How hypertension affects our brain?

Beside heart brain is the other organ that gets most damaged by hypertension. Hypertension causes stroke in brain. Stroke is similar to heart attack.

Stroke is similar to heart attack but occurs in brain. High blood pressure damage the blood vessels that supply blood to deliver oxygen and glucose to brain cells. With damaged or blocked blood vessels brain cells may not receive oxygen or glucose. In turn brain cells may die which is medically termed as Stroke. Also, there may be rupture of vessels due to high blood pressure causing bleeding inside the brain and permanent damage to brain. 40% or more people with stroke has stage 2 hypertension (160/90 mmHg) or more. The risk of stroke is 10 times more with high blood pressure.

A transient ischemic attack (TIA) also called "silent stroke" is another effect of hypertension. In TIA Blood flow to the brain is blocked for a short period of time (less than 15 minutes). TIA gives all the sign of stroke such as loss of consciousness, weakness of limbs, headache and vertigo, but the symptom improves in 24 hours without any treatment. TIA is in reality a warning sign of stroke. And usually if not treated TIA often leads to stroke.

Memory loss, confusion, problems with speaking and understanding is termed as Dementia, It may occur in late part of our life (age 70 or more) caused by untreated hypertension. It happened as high blood pressure damages small blood vessels supplying oxygen to the brain. With damage brain cells, may die and function of brain is hampered. With hypertension, the dementia occurs is called as vascular dementia.

It is a seriously disabling condition.

What are the signs of Stroke?
Unlike TIA or hypertension Stroke shows specific symptoms and sign. If you experience any of the following symptoms you or a loved one could be having a stroke, get help immediately.

- Sudden numbness or weakness in the face, arm, or leg (especially only on one side of the body)
- Sudden loss of vision or decreased vision in one or both eyes
- Sudden paralysis or inability to move part of the body

- Sudden pounding headache with nausea and with vomiting
- Difficulty in speaking, slurring of speech or difficulty understanding simple sentences
- Difficulty swallowing both solid and liquids. Cough when swallowing liquids
- Dizziness, vertigo, loss of balance, or poor coordination
- Brief loss of consciousness with or without convulsion
- Sudden confusion or disorientation

Effect of hypertension on blood vessels?

There are some harmful complications of high blood pressure on your blood vessels. With hypertension or high blood pressure your heart and blood vessels have to work more. As high blood pressure gives extra pressure on your blood vessels specially on arteries It damages your blood vessel walls. They get microscopic tears. These microscopic tear forms scar tissue and over time can form plaque and block the blood flow.

High blood pressure causes the blood vessels to lose its elasticity too.

Effect of hypertension on heart?

Heart is the major organ getting effected by Hypertension or high blood pressure. There is a medical term "Hypertensive heart disease" to describe the effect of hypertension on heart. Studies show hypertension is responsible for 25% of all heart diseases. 68% of heart failure in people over 65 occur for high blood pressure. Women are more effected by heart failure due to hypertension.

Uncontrolled high blood pressure causes structural changes in the heart. By prolonged uncontrolled hypertension there may be thickening of heart muscles (termed as left ventricular hypertrophy). It causes enlargement of heart. Enlarged has a greater chance of failure or attack. Blood vessels supplying oxygen to heart called coronary arteries may become weak or blocked by hypertension, this may lead to heart attack or myocardial infarction.

Is it right to use antihypertensive drugs every other day or 2 - 3 times per week?

NO. Usually the effect of the majority of antihypertensive drugs may last upto 24 hours. So, even drugs whose effect is of the longest duration will not be effective if you take it every other day.

You should take medicines in proper duration to get a beneficial effect from the medicine.

When blood pressure Is high should I take an extra antihypertensive pill?

It seems like common sense to get an extra pill when BP is high but medicines specially blood pressure medicines don't work that way. The treatment for hypertension is different from other condition such as a headache, where you may benefit by taking an extra aspirin. In case of hypertension the use of extra pills when a measurement reveals high levels is completely wrong and could be dangerous for you.

Do not panic if measurement shows a sudden and very high rise in blood pressure. Usually sudden high blood pressure is a temporary rise and the result of a stress related situation. Check blood pressure again after 30 minutes after some rest.

If your blood pressure is still very high consult your doctor. Do not increase or add medicines without consulting your doctor.

What must be done when blood pressure is too low?

The goal of treatment of high blood pressure is to lower systolic pressure below 140 and diastolic pressure below 90; In case of patients with diabetes mellitus or renal disease even lower levels of systolic pressure (below 130) and diastolic pressure (below 80) may be   preferred.

Usually Blood pressure medicines are designed in proper dose not to lower the pressure suddenly. So, if your blood pressure gets low upto systolic below 100 or diastolic below 70 and you do not have any symptoms such as dizziness, vertigo, tremor or feel like fainting you should continue your prescribed medicine. Consulting your doctor for a change of medicine or dose adjustment may be needed.

Stopping your blood pressure medicine suddenly may increase your blood pressure to a dangerous level, so do not stop taking without consulting your doctor.

Are sedatives tranquilizers effective in lowering blood   pressure?

No. It's a common misconception that stress causes hypertension. Yes, stress may raise your blood pressure but it for a very short period of time. Stress may cause other health problem leading to hypertension. So, tranquilizers (or stress medicine) or sedatives (sleep medicine) have to role in treatment of high blood pressure.

Oranges, coffee: do they really affect blood pressure levels?

A common misconception is that oranges increase blood pressure. In reality oranges do not increase blood pressure. On the contrary they are rich in potassium which is useful in high blood pressure especially those under treatment with a specific class of medicine called   diuretics.

Coffee due to caffeine may increase your heart rate and blood pressure temporarily for upto 2 hours after ingestion. Other caffeine containing drinks such as energy drinks can also cause temporary high blood pressure. But if you drink coffee regularly then you become resistant to caffeine and your heart rate or blood pressure do not increase.

Is there any cure for Hypertension?

Till now there is no cure for hypertension. It means that if you are diagnosed with hypertension you will have the condition rest of your life, but you may control it to a normal level with treatment.

With treatment, you will feel no symptoms or complication of hypertension.

In what level, should blood pressure be lowered with treatment?

The normal level of hypertension is individualized. Age, sex, other associated condition such as diabetes, high cholesterol or kidney diseases determine the optimum level of blood pressure for you.

As a general guideline for an elderly person (age 65 or more) blood pressure lower than 140/90 is preferable. In some instance blood pressure below 130/80 is also advised.

When do, Hypertension need treatment

As soon as you are diagnosed with high blood pressure you should start treatment immediately. Your doctor will run some tests to rule out if you have other associated conditions. You will also need an assessment of your heart, kidney and lung functions.

Usually the first line of treatment, starts just after diagnosis. The goal is to modify your lifestyle, food habit and exercise.

When first line does not lower your Blood, you may need to take medicine. Your doctor will select the best drug for your hypertension and monitor your progress and adjust the dose.

When should I call my doctor?

Here are some general guidelines for emergency which needs consultation;

- Consult your doctor if you have symptoms such as feeling faint, fatigue, nausea, shortness of breath, lightheadedness, headache, excessive sweating, problems with vision, or confusion.
- Your blood pressure is 140/90 or higher on two or more occasions.

Consult your doctor Urgently if:

- Your blood pressure is much higher for example 180/110 or higher.

- There is a severe pounding headache.
- Loss or Blurry vision.

Job with Hypertension

With hypertension, certain work and working condition need special attention.

- **Cold work environment**: Working in a very cold environment without proper dress may induce constriction of blood vessels causing the blood pressure to rise.
- **Work stress:** can result in a rise in the blood pressure temporarily. But prolonged stress at work has a harmful effect on your health.
- **Physical demand:** If workload is heavy and work is physically demanding it may raise your blood pressure.
- **Hot and humid work environment:** If the work environment is hot and humid, it may result in excessive sweating and dilation of blood vessels. This cause sudden drop in blood pressure leading to sudden loss of consciousness. Major accidents may happen.
- **Medicines:** Some medicines to control your blood pressure may also cause a sudden drop of blood pressure when you change posture suddenly, causing loss of consciousness. You need to be careful about this condition.
- **Forgetting the medicine:** For busy working schedule, you may forget to take your medicine which may raise your blood pressure to very high level. Take the medications according to prescribed schedule every day. .

  If you miss a dose of blood pressure medicine, do not take a double dose by trying to make up for the missed dose.

Increased dosage taken at a time will cause a sudden drop in blood pressure, or make it very low.

Hypertension may cause complications such as coronary heart disease, heart failure, stroke, renal failure and pathological changes of the arteries in the retina, which may affect working abilities.

How often should a hypertensive person visit the doctor?

Initially after diagnosis you may need to see your doctor every week for 2 to 3 weeks. This is due to confirm your diagnosis and adjust the drug and dose. These visits are also used to rule out other associated conditions such as diabetes or high cholesterol.

After this you may need to visit your doctor every 6 months unless you have symptoms.

If hypertension runs in your family, would you get it too?

If you have a family history of hypertension, then most likely you will develop the condition too. Hypertension has a strong genetic predisposition. The good news is you can take steps to prevent hypertension or avoid it for a long time.

You need to modify your lifestyle, such as;

- Eat a healthy diet, with less fat. Which includes
- Limit sodium (salt) to less than 1500 mg per day.
- Exercise regularly or do physically demanding work.
- Stop Smoking
- Limit alcohol

Does kosher or sea salt has an effect on hypertension?

Chemically kosher salt and sea salt are the same as table salt containing 40 percent sodium. Table salt is a combination of the two minerals sodium (Na) and chloride (Cl).

Kosher or sea salt can increase your blood pressure.

Can you discontinue treatment if there are no symptoms?

If you are prescribed any medicine for your blood pressure, then after taking them your blood pressure usually becomes normal. After measuring normal blood pressure for some time, you may think you do not need medicines anymore. But this is not the case. Hypertension is a chronic condition, once diagnosed you have to continue treatment for the rest of life. Even when you experience no symptoms for a long time. Hypertension in reality does not give any symptoms. It is often called silent killer.

Follow your healthcare professional's recommendations carefully, even if it means taking medication every day for the rest of your life.

Do not stop medicine without talking with your doctor.

Does wine have a positive effect on hypertension?

If you drink alcohol, including wine you need to set limits. Interestingly in some studies moderate drinking as up to two drinks a day for men, one drink for women, has shown a drop-in blood pressure by 2 to 4 points.

But studies have also proven that heavy and regular drinking alcoholic beverages increase blood pressure. Another aspect of alcohol is it may raise your blood pressure suddenly. It can also cause heart failure, stroke and irregular heartbeats.

On the other hand, regular heavy drinking contributes to high triglycerides, cancer, obesity, alcoholism, suicide and accidents, and it can be highly addictive.

Current recommendation of alcohol is to limit consumption to less than two drinks per day for men and one drink per day for women. Generally, "one drink equals a 12-ounce beer, a four-ounce glass of wine, 1.5 ounces of 80-proof liquor, or one ounce of hard liquor (100-proof)".

Is heart rate and blood pressure related?

Heart rate and blood pressure are related but not all the time. In certain situations, like anxiety heart rate may rise along with blood pressure. But in case of patients with high blood pressure the blood pressure stays high even when the heart rate is low.

If your blood pressure is consistently high but your heart rate stays in typical range, the possibility is you have hypertension and need to consult your doctor.

Is Anxiety and Hypertension related?

Studies have shown there is a significant increase in levels of hypertension occur with anxiety. In studies with Bipolar patients show increased anxiety causes a rise in blood pressure. But most of the time this rise is temporary.

Studies also show the rise of blood pressure may be dramatic and sudden which rise with the anxiety level but long term high blood pressure does not relate to anxiety. Problem is these small and sudden rises also causes damage to blood vessels.

So, you need to consult your doctor if there are frequent anxiety attacks.

Are Recreational drugs with Hypertension dangerous?

Some recreational drugs, such as cocaine, ecstasy and amphetamines cause high blood pressure. These drugs work on our brain to make us high. They cause a dramatic increase in your blood pressure and raise your risk of having a stroke or a heart attack. You should avoid Recreational drugs even if you only take them occasionally.

What is the effect of Vape on hypertension?

Vape is a new thing. It is difficult to say the effect of vape on hypertension without study. The effect of nicotine we know, it rises the blood pressure for short period of time. But the long-term effect of other chemicals present in vape and effect of glycerin vapor on lung tissue needs study.

Its best if you avoid vape.

How much Alcohol is safe with Hypertension?

If you have high blood pressure, avoid alcohol or limit alcohol. The maximum alcohol you make take is:

- Two drinks a day for men younger than age 65
- One drink a day for men age 65 and older
- One drink a day for women of any age

One drink is considered as

- In case of beer, 12 ounces (355 milliliters)
- 5 ounces (148 milliliters) in case of wine
- In case of 80 proof distilled spirits 1.5 ounces (44 milliliters)

What is the effect of hypertension on sex?

For men, there is a strong link between sexual problems and hypertension. In case of women it may cause decreased sexual satisfaction.

In case of men

- Erection is achieved by strong blood flow in the spongy part of penile tissue. With uncontrolled and prolonged hypertension damage to these vessels occur. Vessels become hard, less flexible and narrow. This leads to poor erection sometimes erectile dysfunction (inability to achieve an erection).
- Hypertension may also reduce sexual desire. A single episode of erectile dysfunction may cause severe performance anxiety leads men to avoid sex. Sometimes this anxiety itself leads to erectile dysfunction
- Some drugs used to treat hypertension (such as Beta Blocker, Diuretics) causes inability to achieve erection or erectile dysfunction.

A link between high blood pressure and sexual problems is proven in men. For women who have decreased sexual satisfaction, it's not yet proved that high blood pressure is to blame.

In case of women

- The sexual problems of hypertension in women are less pronounced. It may reduce sexual desire, but the mechanism is not well understood.
- Uncontrolled high blood pressure may reduce blood flow to vagina leading to increased vaginal dryness and difficulty achieving orgasm.
- Women also experience anxiety and relationship issues due to sexual dysfunction.

High blood pressure medications that can cause sexual dysfunction as a side effect include:

- Water pills (diuretics). Diuretics decrease blood flow to the penis, making it difficult to achieve an erection.
- Beta blockers. These medications such as propranolol, are associated with sexual dysfunction.

To reduce the risk of sexual problems, take medications exactly as prescribed. Consult your doctor about other possible medications that may have fewer side effects.

Can Erectile Dysfunction occur with Hypertension?

ED means an inability to achieve erection, it is a common problem associated with long term uncontrolled high blood pressure. We achieve erection by increased blood supplied to the spongy part of our penile tissue. High blood pressure that is not properly controlled damages these blood vessels, making it less flexible and narrow. It makes difficult to achieve an erection.

There are many proven treatments you can try. Your doctor has many choices to choose the best one for you. Now we have PDE5 inhibitors, Viagra, Cialis, Levitra, and Staxyn. These drugs work in a similar way, by increasing your blood supply to genital organ. Keep in mind that they do not increase or modify your sexual urges, they make it possible to achieve erection when you are sexually aroused.

No one of them has been proven to work better than the others. But the time they take to start working and the duration of their effects vary. You should consider one based on your sexual habits.

Among these drugs, Viagra works in a short time 15 to 30 minutes and stays active for 2 to 4 hours. Levitra and Cialis becomes active in an hour and stays active longer. Cialis has the longest activity upto 36 hours.

Before trying one of these drugs, you need to consult your doctor.

Can Viagra be used with Hypertension?

Viagra and similar drugs are approved to be taken with hypertension. It is tested and proven to work safely even if you have high blood pressure. But some medication or herbal preparation is dangerous if you take them with Viagra or similar medicines.

Following are some drugs and condition with possible dangerous effect if taken with Viagra or other sexual enhancement drugs;

- Alpha Blocker – do not take alpha blockers (used for hypertension or prostate problems) with Cialis, Levitra, Staxyn, or Viagra.
- Do not take nitrate drugs (used for angina or chest pain) with Cialis, Levitra, Staxyn, or Viagra.
- Avoid Cialis, Levitra, Staxyn, or Viagra if you had a heart attack or stroke in the past six months

- If you have kidney or liver disease Cialis, Levitra, Staxyn, or Viagra is dangerous for you.

Consult Your doctor for high blood pressure with erectile dysfunction, he should be able provide you with a safe and effective medication strategy to address both issues.

Conclusion

High blood pressure leading to life threatening complication is a reality. All the study and data indicate that most of us will get high blood pressure. So, you need to be prepared and start preventive measure as early as possible. I hope after reading this book you can choose a plan that works for you.

Always remember high blood pressure or hypertension is easy to control. And with minimal effort you can Prevent Hypertension.

THE END

Other Books by Dr. Shahriar Mostafa

Diagnosed with Diabetes. Now What!

Smallest Book with Everything You Need to Know

https://www.amazon.com/dp/B01HC0CF26

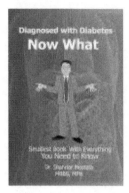

You were living your life to the fullest. Working hard and playing harder. Ignoring symptoms like fatigue, weight loss and increased frequency of urination. Then BAM! Out of the blue you started feeling very sick. You consult with your doctor, he runs some tests and you are diagnosed with diabetes!
Now What!

Should you leave all the things you love to do? Stop eating desserts. Adopt a life of Saints! Should you get panicked and think that's it, this is the end of the road! Well, it's not like that.

This book will help you to keep your diabetes well controlled. It's a small book but packed with information on diabetes you must know. Grab your copy and let's start for a healthy, happy and fulfilling life with Diabetes.

Type One Diabetes:

Smallest book with everything you need to know

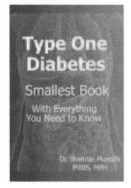

https://www.amazon.com/dp/B01AQOJ21C

As soon as you learn that you or your child has type one diabetes you become terrified. What happens in type one diabetes? What to do to cure it? How to control it? How to explain this to a child? What's causing it? Why did it happen to me? Thousand and thousand questions pop up in your mind. You search the internet which shows a million pages. You ask your health care personal but not satisfied with the answers. You become confused, afraid and angry.

But you don't have to be confused or afraid. You are not alone. Type one diabetes is a common disease. About 350 million people worldwide have diabetes. It is easy to control. It does not keep you from anything the life has to offer. But there is a catch, you have to control type one diabetes all your life.

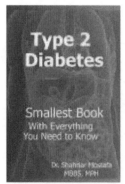

Type 2 Diabetes:

Smallest book with everything you need to know

https://www.amazon.com/dp/B01FUGZASK

Diabetes is a common disease. About 350 million people worldwide have diabetes. It is easy to control. It does not keep you from anything the life has to offer. But there is a catch, you have to control Diabetes all your life.

This book is small and you do not have to read this book from page one to the end. You can start anywhere and slowly finish it. Use the table of contents to find the topic of your interest and start from there. You can finish this book in just 1 hour. In 1 hour, you will have all important information on Type 2 Diabetes. This book will give the confidence, hope and information to live a normal, happy life with Type 2 Diabetes.

Pregnancy & Diabetes:

Smallest Book with Everything You need to know

https://www.amazon.com/dp/B01CEDAH08

If you are pregnant or planning for pregnancy, congratulations. Pregnancy is a life changing event. It takes a lot of courage and a lot
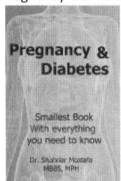
more love to make a decision to have a baby. A lot of planning is also needed before, during and after the pregnancy. Most of us never think twice about diabetes, unless we have it. But diabetes specifically gestational diabetes is a major concern during pregnancy, even if you do not have diabetes.

43480338R00074

Made in the USA
Middletown, DE
10 May 2017